Liver Pathology

Editors

SANJAY KAKAR
DHANPAT JAIN

SURGICAL PATHOLOGY CLINICS

surgpath.theclinics.com

Consulting Editor
JOHN R. GOLDBLUM

June 2013 • Volume 6 • Number 2

ELSEVIER

1600 John F. Kennedy Boulevard • Suite 1800 • Philadelphia, Pennsylvania, 19103-2899

http://www.theclinics.com

SURGICAL PATHOLOGY CLINICS Volume 6, Number 2
June 2013 ISSN 1875-9181, ISBN-13: 978-1-4557-7338-1

Editor: Joanne Husovski

Surgical Pathology Clinics (ISSN 1875-9181) is published quarterly by Elsevier Inc., 360 Park Avenue South, New York, NY 10010. Months of issue are March, June, September, and December. Business and Editorial Office: Elsevier Inc., 1600 John F. Kennedy Blvd., Ste. 1800, Philadelphia, PA 19103-2899. Accounting and Circulation Offices: Elsevier Inc., 3251 Riverport Lane, Maryland Heights, MO 63043. Periodicals postage paid at New York, NY and at additional mailing offices. Subscription prices are $191.00 per year (US individuals), $220.00 per year (US institutions), $94.00 per year (US students/residents), $239.00 per year (Canadian individuals), $249.00 per year (Canadian Institutions), $239.00 per year (foreign individuals), $249.00 per year (foreign institutions), and $116.00 per year (international & Canadian students/residents). Foreign air speed delivery is included in all *Clinics'* subscription prices. All prices are subject to change without notice. **POSTMASTER:** Send address changes to *Surgical Pathology Clinics*, Elsevier, 3251 Riverport Lane, Maryland Heights, MO 63043. Customer Service: 1-800-654-2452 (US). From outside the United States, call 1-314-447-8871. Fax: 1-314-447-8029. E-mail: JournalsCustomerServiceusa@elsevier.com (for print support) and JournalsOnlineSupport-usa@elsevier.com (for online support).

Reprints. For copies of 100 or more, of articles in this publication, please contact the Commercial Reprints Department, Elsevier Inc., 360 Park Avenue South, New York, NY 10010-1710. Tel. (212) 633-3812; Fax: (212) 462-1935; E-mail: reprints@elsevier.com.

Contributors

CONSULTING EDITOR

JOHN R. GOLDBLUM, MD
Chairman, Professor of Pathology, Department
of Anatomic Pathology, Cleveland Clinics
Lerner College of Medicine, Cleveland Clinic,
Cleveland, Ohio

EDITORS

SANJAY KAKAR, MD
Benedict Yen Endowed Professor of
Pathology, University of California,
San Francisco, Chief of Pathology,
VA Medical Center, San Francisco, California

DHANPAT JAIN, MD
Professor of Pathology, Director, GI and
Liver Pathology, Department of Pathology,
Yale University School of Medicine,
New Haven, Connecticut

AUTHORS

PIERRE BEDOSSA, MD, PhD
Department of Pathology, Beaujon Hospital
and Clichy University Denis Diderot, Paris,
France

CRISTINA D. COLE, MD
Resident Pathologist, Indiana University
School of Medicine Indianapolis, Indiana

GUADALUPE GARCIA-TSAO, MD
Section of Digestive Diseases, Department of
Medicine, Yale University School of Medicine,
New Haven, Connecticut

RYAN M. GILL, MD, PhD
Assistant Professor, Department of Pathology,
University of California, San Francisco,
San Francisco, California

ALLEN M. GOWN, MD
PhenoPath Laboratories, Seattle, Washington

DHANPAT JAIN, MD
Professor of Pathology, Director, GI and
Liver Pathology, Department of Pathology,
Yale University School of Medicine, New
Haven, Connecticut

SANJAY KAKAR, MD
Benedict Yen Endowed Professor of
Pathology, University of California,
San Francisco, Chief of Pathology,
VA Medical Center, San Francisco, California

CHARLES R. LASSMAN, MD, PhD
Professor, Department of Pathology and
Laboratory Medicine, David Geffen School of
Medicine at UCLA, Los Angeles, California

ESMERALDA CELIA MARGINEAN, MD
Associate Professor, Department of Pathology,
The Ottawa Hospital, Ottawa University,
Ottawa, Ontario, Canada

RAFFAELLA A. MOROTTI, MD
Department of Pathology, Yale University
School of Medicine, New Haven, Connecticut

BITA V. NAINI, MD
Assistant Professor, Department of Pathology
and Laboratory Medicine, David Geffen School
of Medicine at UCLA, Los Angeles, California

VALÉRIE PARADIS, MD, PhD
Department of Pathology, Beaujon Hospital,
Clichy, Paris, France

ROMIL SAXENA, MBBS, MD, FRCPATH (UK)
Professor of Pathology and Laboratory
Medicine, Professor of Medicine, Indiana
University School of Medicine Indianapolis,
Indiana

NAFIS SHAFIZADEH, MD
Staff Pathologist, Southern California
Permanente Medical Group, Woodland
Hills Medical Center, Woodland Hills,
California

Contents

are acute cellular rejection, late acute rejection (centrizonal/parenchymal rejection), chronic rejection, plasma cell hepatitis, idiopathic posttransplant chronic hepatitis, fibrosing cholestatic hepatitis, selected viral infections (cytomegalovirus, Epstein-Barr virus, and hepatitis E), and acute antibody-mediated rejection.

WHO recognized variants of scirrhous HCC, fibrolamellar carcinoma, combined HCC-cholangiocarcinoma (HCC-CC), sarcomatoid HCC, undifferentiated carcinoma, and lymphoepithelioma-like HCC are discussed in detail. Other subtypes including clear cell HCC, diffuse cirrhosis-like HCC, steatohepatitic HCC, transitional liver cell tumor, and CAP carcinoma are also reviewed.

SURGICAL PATHOLOGY CLINICS

Preface
Liver Pathology: Unraveling the Art of Pattern Recognition

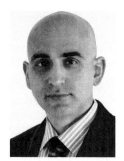
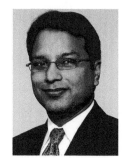

Sanjay Kakar, MD   Dhanpat Jain, MD

Editors

The liver was regarded as the "seat" of emotions, courage, and even the soul by several ancient civilizations. As knowledge of anatomy and physiology evolved, this exalted status was usurped by other organs like the heart and the brain. Despite these setbacks, the liver has been held in awe by writers, poets, philosophers, scientists, and the like. Shakespeare happily subscribed to the notion of the liver as the source of strength and immortalized phrases like "liver as white as milk" (cowardly, *Twelfth Night*) and "lily-livered boys" (frightened soldiers, *King Lear*). In the contemporary era, the liver continues to inspire and enthrall a new breed of artists, who have a penchant for pattern recognition and are happy hunting a myriad of fascinating features hiding in the nooks and corners of portal tracts and lobules in liver biopsies. These artists marvel at hematoxylin and eosin–stained sections and amalgamate the plethora of colors presented by a waltz of special stains to identify patterns, a necessary step to unlock the intricacies of liver disease that are often naively oversimplified as "elevated LFTs."

There have been significant advances in immunohistochemistry and molecular techniques, but the critical evaluation of hematoxylin and eosin–stained slides remains the basis of liver biopsy evaluation, especially in the nonneoplastic setting. This volume of *Surgical Pathology Clinics* highlights selected topics in liver pathologic abnormality that have seen many advances in recent years and frequently pose diagnostic challenges. The articles on steatohepatitis, autoimmune diseases/overlap syndromes, and liver allograft pathology abnormality highlight the conceptual and diagnostic challenges in these areas. The significance of different combinations of morphologic features in different clinicopathologic settings is discussed. The article on regression of cirrhosis emphasizes that we have moved past the era of "fact versus fantasy" debate of fibrosis regression in the liver. Further classification of cirrhosis into clinically meaningful subgroups is also discussed. The series also includes a review of pediatric cholestatic disorders, a particularly challenging area where identification of various genetic mutations affecting proteins involved in bile synthesis or transport has led to recognition of a variety of disorders that were otherwise lumped as "neonatal hepatitis." The terminology of these disorders and their differentiation from one another remain a challenge even for experts in the field.

The neoplastic section provides the reader a foray into the WHO classification of hepatocellular adenomas and the practical use of immunohistochemistry to identify these subtypes. The question of primary versus metastatic tumor is perhaps the most commonly encountered situation in the clinical practice of liver pathology. A detailed analysis of currently available immunohistochemical markers and suggestions for their judicious use in diverse clinical settings are provided. Hepatocellular

Surgical Pathology 6 (2013) ix–x
http://dx.doi.org/10.1016/j.path.2013.03.009
1875-9181/13/$ – see front matter © 2013 Published by Elsevier Inc.

surgpath.theclinics.com

x

carcinoma comes in several well-disguised forms and can be mistaken for glandular, neuroendocrine, and even nonepithelial tumors like melanoma and angiomyolipoma. The last article focuses on the histologic variants of hepatocellular carcinoma to enable a correct diagnosis even in the face of atypical histologic and immunohistochemical features, facilitating appropriate treatment with surgery, chemotherapy, and/or transplantation.

In the spirit of the history of this series, the articles are embellished with images, tables, and summaries that illustrate salient features and help distinguish entities from close mimics. We hope that this issue will provide updates on selected topics and serve as a guide to handle practical problems of liver pathology evaluation in daily practice. We express our sincere gratitude to the authors for the effort in sharing their expertise despite overcommitted schedules. We are also grateful to Dr John Goldblum, consulting editor, for conferring this guest editorial opportunity on us. Special thanks are also due to Joanne Husovski of Elsevier, whose efficiency and perseverance were instrumental in molding the text into its final shape.

Sanjay Kakar, MD
Benedict Yen Endowed Professor of Pathology
University of California, San Francisco
Chief of Pathology
VA Medical Center
San Francisco, CA 94121, USA

Dhanpat Jain, MD
Professor
Director of GI and Liver Pathology
Department of Pathology
Yale University School of Medicine
New Haven, CT 06520, USA

E-mail addresses:
sanjay.kakar@ucsf.edu (S. Kakar)
Dhanpat.Jain@yale.edu (D. Jain)

Pediatric Cholestatic Disorders
Approach to Pathologic Diagnosis

Raffaella A. Morotti, MD*, Dhanpat Jain, MD

KEYWORDS

- Pediatric cholestatic disorders • Cholestatic jaundice • Neonatal cholestasis
- Pediatric liver disease

ABSTRACT

This article addresses select liver diseases that are commonly seen in the pediatric group and pose diagnostic challenges in practice. The key genetic/molecular abnormalities, clinical features, histopathologic findings, diagnostic modalities, differential diagnoses, and possible pitfalls in diagnosis are discussed in detail. Although recent advances in understanding the pathophysiology of bile synthesis and transport along with advances in molecular genetics have allowed a better characterization of many of these liver diseases, significant overlap in the histopathologic features of many of these disorders still leads to diagnostic challenges for the pathologist.

OVERVIEW

Cholestatic disorders in the pediatric age differ from cholestatic disorders in adults. Cholestatic jaundice usually is a later finding in adult liver disease, whereas it is a common presentation of liver disease in neonates and infants. This is likely related to the immaturity of hepatic excretory function, which results in the greater number of cholestatic liver disorders in the neonatal period than later in life.

Cholestatic jaundice is clinically defined by an increase in the level of conjugated bilirubin. Accepted guidelines define abnormal conjugated bilirubin values as greater than 1 mg/dL when the total bilirubin is less than 5 mg/dL or if it represents more than 20% of the total bilirubin when the total bilirubin is greater than 5 mg/dL.[1]

The remarkable progress in the past 30 years of our understanding of the pathophysiology of bile synthesis and transport, along with advances in molecular genetics, has allowed characterization of a subset of liver diseases that present in neonates and infants. As a result, the diagnosis of neonatal hepatitis (also known as idiopathic neonatal hepatitis of unknown etiology or giant cell hepatitis), which formerly represented more than 65% of neonatal and infantile cholestatic diseases, has now decreased to 15%. The common cholestatic diseases of neonates and infants include the following[2]:

- Biliary atresia: 25%–30%
- Bile salt synthesis and transport defects: 25%
- Other metabolic diseases: 20%
- Idiopathic neonatal hepatitis: 15%
- Alpha-1-antitripsin (A1AT) deficiency: 10%
- Viral infections: 5%

See **Fig. 1** for a simplified diagnostic approach for neonatal cholestasis.

The common causes of neonatal cholestasis can be broadly divided into 2 groups:

1. *Obstructive* (biliary) cholestasis, which includes biliary atresia, choledochal cysts, bile duct paucity, neonatal sclerosing cholangitis, cystic fibrosis, and gallstones.
2. *Intrahepatic* cholestasis, which includes various viral and bacterial infections, genetic/metabolic disorders, endocrine disorders, toxic or drug mediated, and parenteral nutrition.

Microscopically, pediatric cholestatic disorders also differ from those in adults. Some histopathologic features, such as giant cell transformation of hepatocytes and bile duct paucity, are more frequently seen in neonatal liver disorders than in

Department of Pathology, Yale University School of Medicine, 310 Cedar Street, PO Box 208023, New Haven, CT 06520-8023, USA
* Corresponding author.
E-mail address: raffaella.morotti@yale.edu

Surgical Pathology 6 (2013) 205–225
http://dx.doi.org/10.1016/j.path.2013.03.001
1875-9181/13/$ – see front matter © 2013 Elsevier Inc. All rights reserved.

surgpath.theclinics.com

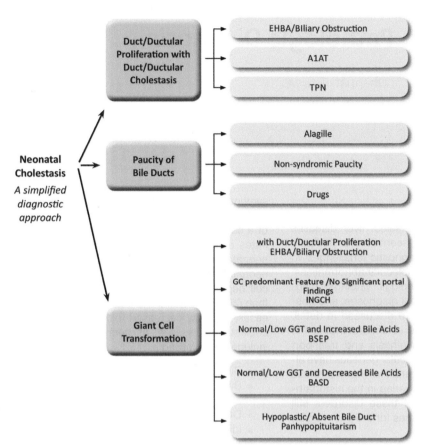

Fig. 1. Simplified diagnostic approach to the neonatal cholestastis. INGCH, idiopathic neonatal giant cell hepatitis.

Neonatal Cholestasis
A simplified diagnostic approach

Duct/Ductular Proliferation with Duct/Ductular Cholestasis
- EHBA/Biliary Obstruction
- A1AT
- TPN

Paucity of Bile Ducts
- Alagille
- Non-syndromic Paucity
- Drugs

Giant Cell Transformation
- with Duct/Ductular Proliferation EHBA/Biliary Obstruction
- GC predominant Feature /No Significant portal Findings INGCH
- Normal/Low GGT and Increased Bile Acids BSEP
- Normal/Low GGT and Decreased Bile Acids BASD
- Hypoplastic/ Absent Bile Duct Panhypopituitarism

adults; however, they are not specific for any particular etiologic subgroup. Frequently, obstructive and hepatic features show a significant overlap. Duct/ductular proliferation may be seen associated with portal/lobular inflammation, making the identification of the underlying etiology more complex. Type and location of cholestasis is also fairly nonspecific. Thus, a combination of findings, rather than a single feature, is often more helpful in the differential diagnosis, and correlation with clinical features, laboratory parameters, and genetic testing is essential to arrive at the correct diagnosis. This article is largely devoted to the diagnostic approach to the most common cholestatic disorders that are unique to children, particularly in the early neonatal/infantile period. **Table 1** depicts a simplified approach to the diagnosis of the main

cholestatic diseases of early pediatric age in relation to the distinctive histologic feature.

EXTRAHEPATIC BILIARY ATRESIA

Extrahepatic biliary atresia (EHBA) defines stenosis or atresia of the extrahepatic biliary tree. The incidence of EHBA varies from 1 in 18,000 live births in Europe and North America to 1 in 5000 in Taiwan. It is the most common cause of cholestasis in the newborn, representing approximately 25% of neonatal cholestasis cases and has remained unchanged over the years. It is the most common indication for liver transplantation in children. The pathogenesis is unknown and presumed to be the result of a variety of predisposing insults.[3]

Table 1
Comparison of prevalence of histologic features in cholestatic disease of infancy

	EHBA	TPNAC	Syndromic Paucity	A1AT	PFIC 1,2,3	BASD	NGCH
Duct/ductular proliferation	+++	+++	Rarely	Rarely	In PFIC3	No	No
Duct paucity	With advanced disease	Younger infants	By definition but occasionally present early in disease	++	In PFIC2 occasionally	No	In panhypopituitarism
Giant cell	++	++	±	±	++ (PFIC2)	+++	+++
Cholestasis	Ductular Hepatocellular Canalicular	Ductular Hepatocellular Canalicular	Hepatocellular Canalicular Ductular	Hepatocellular Canalicular Ductular	Hepatocellular Canalicular Ductular	Ductular Hepatocellular	Canalicular Hepatocellular
Steatosis	Yes	Yes	No	No	No	No	No
Portal inflammation	Neutrophilic pericholangitis EMH	Neutrophilic pericholangitis EMH	Rarely	Rarely	In PFIC2 and PFIC3	Yes	Variable Lymphocytic EMH
Lobular inflammation	No	No	No	No	In PFIC3	+	Variable
Iron deposition	No	No	No	No	No	5βRD ZS	Described
Fibrosis	Portal Bridging Cirrhosis	Portal Bridging Perivenular Cirrhosis	Portal Non-uniform bridging Cirrhosis	Portal Bridging Cirrhosis	Portal Portal to central bridging Cirrhosis	Portal Bridging Cirrhosis	Portal Bridging Pericellular

Abbreviations: 5βRD, 5β reductase deficiency; A1AT, alpha-1-antitrypsin; BASD, bile acid synthesis disorder; EHBA, extrahepatic biliary atresia; EMH, extramedullary hematopoiesis; NGCH, neonatal giant cell hepatitis; PFIC, progressive familial intrahepatic cholestasis; TPNAC, total parenteral nutrition associated cholestasis.

The clinical presentation is usually within the first 2 months of life, with obstructive-type jaundice (direct hyperbilirubinemia), acholic (pale) stools, dark urine, increased alkaline phosphatases and gamma glutamyltransferase (GGT), and variable increases in aminotransferases.

Anatomically, 3 main types of EHBA are described:

1. Type 1 (5%), in which the obstruction is at the level of the common bile duct and is usually associated with proximal cystic dilatation.
2. Type 2 (2%), in which the obstruction is at the level of the common hepatic duct, with patent ducts at the porta hepatis.
3. Type 3 (>95%), in which the obstruction is the more proximal at the porta hepatis level. In subtype 3a, a hypoplastic gallbladder and portion of the common bile duct can be patent. Approximately 20% are associated with other congenital malformations; the most common is biliary atresia/splenic malformation syndrome, including polysplenia, situs inversus, and vascular anomalies.

Clinically, 2 types of EHBA are identified:

1. Embryonal or syndromic form: 30%
2. Perinatal or acquired form: 70%

There is no histopathological distinction between these 2 groups.[4] Jaundice usually develops from ages 3 to 6 weeks in an otherwise thriving infant. In the embryonal form, cholestatic jaundice may be present from birth.

The diagnosis of biliary atresia is time sensitive, as the best success to obtain bile flow occurs when the hepatic portoenterostomy/Kasai procedure (HPE) is done before 60 to 90 days of age.[5] Some investigators, however, suggest that the degree of liver fibrosis, independent of age, is the major determinant of outcome.[6]

HISTOLOGIC FINDINGS

A liver biopsy can correctly predict extrahepatic biliary obstruction in more than 90% of cases, directing the evaluation toward cholangiography.[7] Accuracy of the pathologic diagnosis ranges from 79% to 98%, and some consider histopathology to be the gold standard for the diagnosis of biliary atresia.[8,9]

The histopathology findings may be divided into portal and lobular changes.

Portal Changes

Portal changes include ductal and/or ductular proliferation and cholestasis with bile plugs in ducts and canaliculi, and sometimes can mimic a ductal plate malformation (**Fig. 2**A–C). Duct proliferation and bile plugs are considered the best predictors of obstruction.[7] The intralobular bile ducts may appear injured and portal tract edema and fibrosis are variable. Florid ductular proliferation is frequently accompanied by a neutrophilic reaction (pericholangitis). Loss of intralobular bile ducts is more frequently seen later in the disease.

Lobular Changes

Lobular changes include hepatocellular, cholestasis, giant cell transformation, and a variable amount of extramedullary hematopoiesis. Giant cell transformation is seen in approximately 20% to 50% of patients,[4,10] but is never as prominent as it is in neonatal hepatitis. With progression, other features of chronic cholestasis, which include cholate stasis, copper deposition in periportal hepatocytes, and Mallory hyaline, also become evident.

Progressive fibrosis results in biliary cirrhosis in about 1 to 6 months. Sinusoidal fibrosis is typically absent and fibrosis is largely portal based, which eventually evolves into cirrhosis. Cirrhosis has the typical characteristics of biliary-type cirrhosis with large fibrous bands, portal-to-portal bridging, and extensive duct/ductular proliferation. The fibrosis can form a geographic pattern and central venules may still be preserved in many cirrhotic nodules. Geographic fibrosis and ductular proliferation, mimicking ductal plate malformation, can be seen, especially after Kasai portoenterostomy (see **Fig. 2**D, E). Patients with the syndromic form of EHBA may present with cirrhosis at a younger age; on the other hand, older infants with the "late" acquired form of biliary atresia may not have cirrhosis. Hepatocellular carcinoma in association with EHBA has been reported, especially after HPE.[11]

DIFFERENTIAL DIAGNOSIS IN EHBA

Clinically and pathologically, the major differentiation is from various entities that are included under the neonatal hepatitis group, as the management differs. The key points for the diagnosis of EHBA are summarized in **Box 1**. The 2 conditions, which can histologically mimic biliary atresia very closely, include total parenteral nutrition (TPN)-associated cholestasis and A1AT deficiency. Both disorders histologically may show features suggestive of obstruction with variable ductular reaction, and their differentiation may be impossible without access to clinical data. The key features in the differential diagnosis are shown in **Table 2**. Neonatal primary sclerosing cholangitis is a rare entity whose recognition as a distinct entity is debated (see later in this article).

Fig. 2. (*A*) Example of EHBA showing marked ductal proliferation and giant cell reaction (*arrow*) (H&E, 100×). (*B*) Example of EHBA showing irregular ductular profiles, reminiscent of ductal-plate malformation with intraluminal structure with circular configuration around a fibrovascular core. Extramedullary hematopoiesis is present (*arrow*) (H&E 400×). (*C*) Ductular (*large arrow*) and canalicular cholestasis (*small arrow*) (H&E 200×).

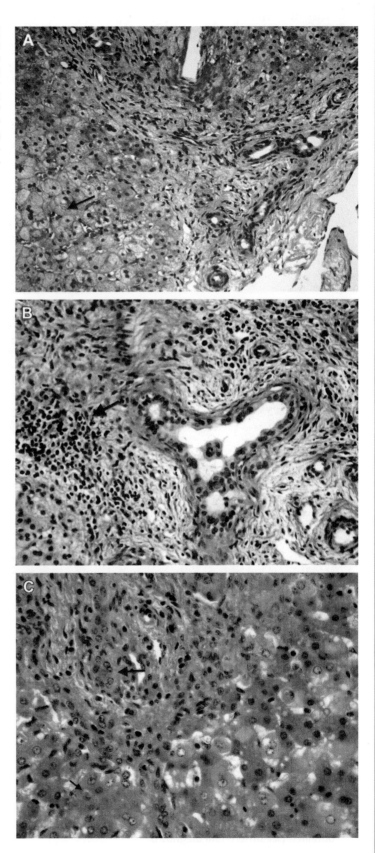

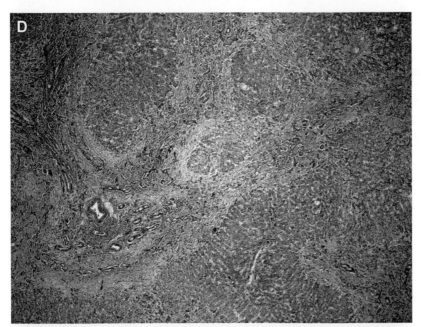

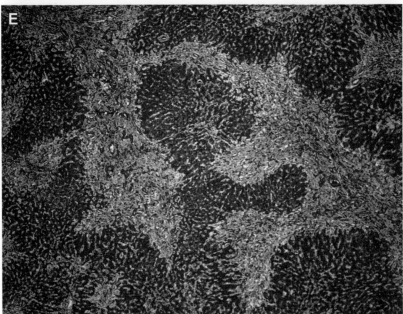

Fig. 2. (*D*) Explanted liver with EHBA after Kasai HPE with extensive ductular proliferation, ductal cholestasis, bridging fibrosis, and cirrhosis. Ductular proliferation as seen here can mimic ductal plate malformation (H&E 100×). (*E*) Explanted liver after Kasai HPE, highlighting geographic fibrosis and irregular profile of proliferating ductules mimicking congenital hepatic fibrosis (Trichrome stain, 100×).

Box 1
Key points: extrahepatic biliary atresia

1. Most frequent cholestatic disease of the neonatal period, amenable to surgical correction. Kasai portoenterostomy has possibly better results if performed at not later than 3 months of age. Diagnosis is time sensitive.

2. Pathologic diagnosis is not definitive, but should be able to exclude most of nonsurgically correctable causes of neonatal liver cholestasis, and lead to surgical exploration for confirmation of the diagnosis.

3. Histologic findings more reliable for this diagnosis are ductal/ductular proliferation and ductal/ductular cholestasis (bile plugs).

4. Clinical data to rule out cholestatic diseases that can mimic on histologic ground EHBA should be obtained (see differential diagnosis).

Table 2
Extrahepatic biliary atresia differential diagnosis

EHBA vs	Distinguishing Features
1. A1AT	Duct paucity is more frequently seen in A1AT Ductal/ductular proliferation is more indicative of obstruction, but can be seen in A1AT Classical PAS-D–resistant inclusions are not always seen in neonates and clinical correlation is mandatory
2. PNALD	Same features, clinical correlation is mandatory
3. Idiopathic NGCH	Occasionally EHBA may have a prominent lobular giant cell reaction. Portal findings of ductal/ductular proliferation should be considered in favor of an obstructive process.

Abbreviations: A1AT, alpha-1-antitrypsin; EHBA, extrahepatic biliary atresia; NGCH, neonatal giant cell hepatitis; PAS-D, periodic acid-Schiff diastase; PNALD, parenteral nutrition associated liver disease.

PITFALLS IN EHBA

Diagnostic pitfalls are related to fragmentation of the biopsy or an insufficient amount of portal tracts to evaluate. If the biopsy is performed before 8 weeks of age, the histology may not show all of the typical findings.

PARENTERAL NUTRITION–ASSOCIATED LIVER DISEASE

Parenteral nutrition (PN) may be associated with cholestasis (PNAC) and may progress to severe liver disease (PNALD). In neonates and infants, the risk factors associated with PNAC include prematurity, low birth weight, necrotizing enterocolitis, and sepsis, although none is reported as an independent risk factor. The pathogenesis of the disease is unknown, likely multifactorial, and possibly related to the immaturity of the bile excretory system.

Cholestasis may appear within 2 weeks of PN and cirrhosis may develop as early as 3 months of therapy. Duration of PN is an important predictor for developing PNAC and its severity. The elevation of liver enzymes does not consistently reflect the severity of the liver disease.[12]

HISTOLOGIC FINDINGS

Hepatocytic and canalicular cholestasis are the most frequent and earliest histologic findings (Fig. 3A). Mild ductular reaction and ductal cholestasis can be seen after a few weeks, and become prominent with disease progression (see Fig. 3B). Portal edema may be present, as in cholestasis of obstructive etiology (see Fig. 3C). Periportal inflammation may be seen and giant cell transformation is reported in about one-third of cases.[13] Paucity of bile ducts has been reported after a short period of PN; however, it should be considered that the number of ducts per portal tract may be fewer in premature neonates. Steatosis is more common in older children and adults compared with infants, but occasionally can be seen with short-term PN. The severity of portal fibrosis correlates with the duration of PN and it can regress after discontinuation of PN. Liver explants with PNALD show perivenular fibrosis in association with severe portal fibrosis, which appears to be characteristic.[14] Cirrhosis is usually micronodular of biliary type. Hepatocellular carcinoma has been reported with prolonged PN use.[15]

DIFFERENTIAL DIAGNOSIS

Histologic findings, particularly ductular proliferation and ductal/ductular cholestasis, are similar to EHBA and differentiation from other biliary disorders can be very difficult; however, with a history of PN, the diagnosis is straightforward. Diagnostic difficulty may arise when PN is associated with another cholestatic disorder, for example, cystic fibrosis (see Fig. 3D) or A1AT deficiency. Careful clinical correlation is required in such situations.

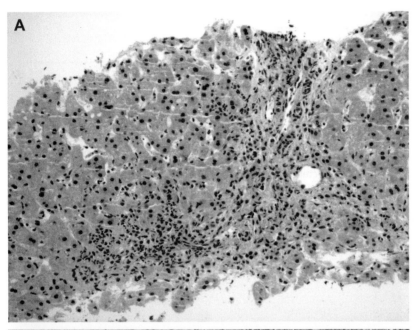

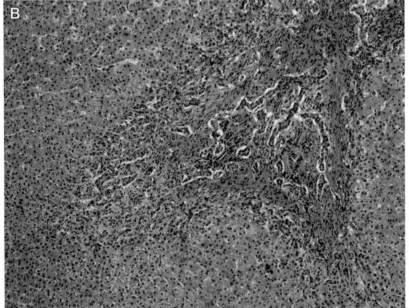

Fig. 3. (*A*) TPN-associated cholestasis, in a 15-year-old child on TPN for 8 weeks. Florid ductular proliferation and mild portal fibrosis (H&E 200×). (*B*) TPN-associated cholestasis showing ductular proliferation and ductular cholestasis can appear similar to EHBA. Portal fibrosis progresses with duration of TPN (H&E 100×).

Fig. 3. (*C*) High power image of a portal tract showing presence of portal tract edema and mild inflammation (Trichrome stain, 400×). (*D*) TPN-associated cholestasis in a patient with cystic fibrosis. In addition to ductular proliferation and ductular cholestasis, paler amorphous secretions typical of cystic fibrosis are present (H&E 200×).

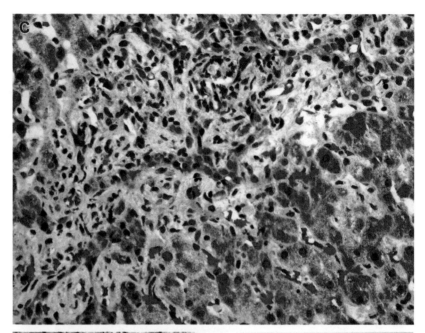

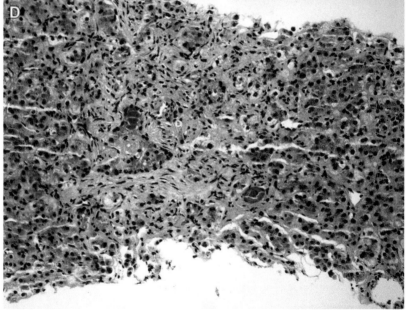

SCLEROSING CHOLANGITIS

Pediatric sclerosing cholangitis (SC) is divided into 4 main groups[16]:

1. Neonatal SC, a genetic disease, is transmitted by autosomal recessive inheritance.
2. Autoimmune SC, or AIH/SC overlap syndrome, is an autoimmune disease usually seen in children and may be associated with inflammatory bowel disease (IBD).
3. SC without autoimmune features has an unknown etiology.
4. SC that is secondary to other diseases, mainly Langerhans cell histiocytosis and immunodeficiencies.

Neonatal SC mimics EHBA with presentation in the first 2 weeks of life and is indistinguishable on liver histology.

The diagnosis rests on cholangiography showing patency of the extrahepatic bile ducts and the

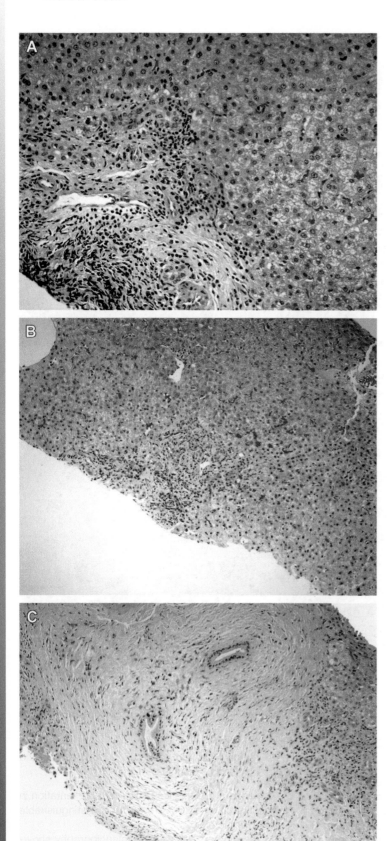

Fig. 4. (*A*) Primary sclerosing cholangitis (PSC) overlap in a 6-year-old child with ulcerative colitis. Portal tract with interface hepatitis with many plasma cells (H&E 200×). (*B*) Same patient as in *A*, with ductular proliferation in portal tracts (H&E, 100×), and (*C*) large bile duct with irregular lumen, surrounded by concentric fibrosis (H&E, 200×).

characteristic beaded appearance and irregular profiles of the intrahepatic bile ducts.

Overlap syndrome of AIH and SC occurs more frequently in children than in adults and is characterized by both disorders occurring simultaneously or within a short interval. Similar to adults, SC in children is frequently associated with IBD, mainly ulcerative colitis (Fig. 4).

A variant of SC seen in children, defined as small-duct SC, is reported to have the same clinical, biochemical, and histopathological features as "large-duct" SC but with normal cholangiography. This variant is more frequently associated with Crohn disease in children.[17]

PAUCITY OF BILE DUCTS

Paucity of bile ducts is divided into 2 groups, with the syndromic variant referring to Alagille syndrome, and the nonsyndromic type associated with multiple etiologies (Box 2).

Alagille syndrome is an autosomal dominant disease with intrahepatic paucity of bile ducts associated with the following:

- Heart and vascular abnormalities: tetralogy of Fallot, peripheral pulmonary stenosis

---

Box 2
Nonsyndromic bile duct paucity

- Prematurity
- Infection
  - Congenital cytomegalovirus
  - Congenital rubella
  - Congenital syphilis
- Genetic
  - Trisomy 21
  - Trisomy 18
- Metabolic
  - A1AT deficiency
  - PFIC 1 and 2
  - Zellweger syndrome
- Other
  - Late-stage EHBA
  - Graft-versus-host disease
  - Drug (antibiotics)
  - SC
  - Panhypopituitarism

- Spinal abnormality: butterfly vertebrae
- Ocular abnormality: posterior embryotoxon
- Facial irregularity: triangular face
- Renal abnormalities: cystic dysplasia

Approximately 95% have mutations of the *Jagged1* gene and about 1% have mutations of the *Notch2* gene. These genes are located on the long arm of chromosome 20. Infants present with jaundice, debilitating pruritus, increased total and direct bilirubin, and often high GGT. Cholesterol and bile acid levels also are quite elevated. Hepatomegaly is common, with one-third of patients developing portal hypertension and eventually end-stage liver disease. Most infants with Alagille syndrome present for evaluation of hepatic dysfunction. Diagnosis is made by a combination of bile duct paucity in the liver biopsy and at least 3 of 5 major criteria:

1. Cholestasis
2. Heart murmur
3. Embryotoxon
4. Butterfly vertebrae
5. Typical triangular facies

HISTOLOGIC FINDINGS

Paucity of bile ducts refers to a reduced number of interlobular (small) bile ducts. The normal ratio of bile ducts to portal tracts is between 0.9 and 1.8. Paucity may be evaluated as a percentage of portal tracts without bile ducts. Normally this is estimated at 10% to 15% and abnormal (paucity) from 30% to 100%. These values apply to infants born at term (>38 weeks' gestation) and premature infants typically have a lower ratio. Between 33 and 38 weeks of gestation, the bile ducts can be absent in about 40% of portal tracts. An adequate number of portal tracts is required for the evaluation of paucity in a liver biopsy and the recommended minimum number is 10 portal tracts.[18] Liver biopsies from newborns, however, are usually small, and 5 portal tracts have been reported sufficient for the diagnosis.[19] With disease progression, a paucity of portal tracts also can occur.

The histologic findings vary by the age of the patient and progression of the disease. The duct paucity may not be evident in early biopsies and can develop later (usually by 6 months) (Fig. 5). Lobular cholestasis is present and ductular proliferation can be occasionally seen in early biopsies, but is usually absent. Features of nonspecific neonatal hepatitis can be seen in the first month of life.[20] In early biopsies, the changes may range from bile duct injury and duct sclerosis to duct loss. Fibrosis is described

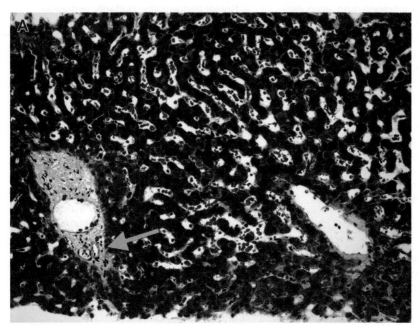

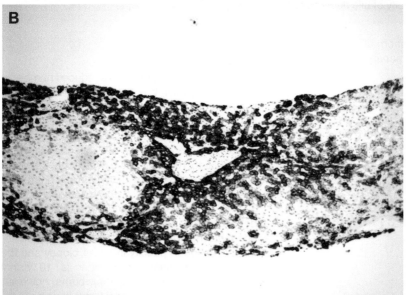

Fig. 5. (*A*) Alagille syndrome showing a portal tract with small artery (*arrow*) and vein and no bile duct (Trichrome stain, 200×). (*B*) Prominent biliary metaplasia of periportal hepatocytes as highlighted by CK7 immunostain. Also note that portal tract lack bile ducts, which can also be seen with a CK19 stain.

as patchy and the progression to cirrhosis appears slower than in other cholestatic diseases. Bridging fibrosis in explanted livers is more commonly seen than full-blown cirrhosis. Hepatocellular carcinomas in patients with Alagille syndrome have been described.[21]

DIFFERENTIAL DIAGNOSIS

Paucity of bile ducts should prompt an investigation to rule out syndromic and nonsyndromic subtypes. In cases with ductular proliferation, the main differential diagnosis is biliary atresia. Additional confounding factors include biliary atresia associated with cardiac abnormalities and failure to visualize the gallbladder by ultrasound, which may incorrectly suggest biliary atresia. Genetic testing of the *Jagged1* gene is commercially available and can confirm the diagnosis in approximately 95% of cases.

A1AT DEFICIENCY

A1AT deficiency is the most common cause of genetic liver disease in childhood. The liver disease is associated almost exclusively with the PiZZ phenotype in children. The usual Pi (protease inhibitor) MM phenotype is associated with normal serum A1AT concentrations in the range of 1.5 to 3.5 g/L by standard determinations. The PiZZ is the classic deficient variant, which in the homozygous state determines a markedly decreased serum concentration of A1AT.

Overt liver disease in children with A1AT deficiency occurs in 10% to 20% of children. The typical clinical presentation is with neonatal cholestasis, acholic stools, hepatomegaly, and increase in serum transaminases. In most cases, the symptoms spontaneously regress by age 6 months. Cirrhosis develops in 20% to 30% of infants who present with neonatal cholestasis and can be seen in the first 6 month of age or later.

HISTOLOGIC FINDINGS

The hepatic histologic features vary depending on the age of the patient. Eosinophilic hyaline globules in the hepatocytes that are positive with periodic acid-Schiff (PAS) stain and diastase resistant (PAS-D) remain the hallmark of the disease, but they are not entirely specific and may not be seen in the first 3 months of life. Instead, a fine granular cytoplasm may be seen, which can be highlighted with PAS-D stain and A1AT immunostain (**Fig. 6**A). One has to be careful when interpreting the A1AT immunostain, as normal hepatocytes also make A1AT and show diffuse cytoplasmic staining, and one needs to look for staining of the granules or the inclusions. When present, the globules are usually multiple, round, homogeneously pink, and located in the periportal hepatocytes (see **Fig. 6**B). They may vary in size up to 40 μm in diameter. The largest are usually encircled by a halo, probably due to a cracking artifact. The globules represent accumulation of abnormal A1AT. By electron microscopy, electron-dense material filling the rough endoplasmic reticulum is characteristic (see **Fig. 6**C).

Besides the globules, the liver histology varies considerably, and may show damaged bile ducts, ductular proliferation, duct paucity, ductular cholestasis and pseudorosettes, giant cell transformation of hepatocytes, portal mononuclear infiltrate, and mild fibrosis. Cirrhosis may develop as early as 6 months of age and can be micronodular or macronodular. Variable amounts of cholestasis, steatosis, and inflammation can be seen. The diagnosis is established with serum levels and phenotyping of the A1AT allele. Hepatocellular and cholangiocarcinoma are known complications.[22,23]

PROGRESSIVE INTRAHEPATIC FAMILIAL CHOLESTASIS

Progressive familial intrahepatic cholestasis (PFIC) is a group of autosomal recessive disorders that usually present in infancy, childhood, or rarely in adults. Three forms have been recognized, in the past called PFIC 1 to 3, and recently renamed after the involved gene as FIC1 deficiency, BSEP (bile salt export pump) deficiency, and MDR3 deficiency, respectively. The most distinctive genetic, clinical, and histologic features of PFIC 1, 2, and 3 are summarized in **Table 3**.

FIC1 DEFICIENCY (FORMERLY PFIC1)

FIC1 deficiency and benign recurrent intrahepatic cholestasis are caused by mutation of the *ATP8B1* gene encoding the FIC1. The most severe form of the disease has been called Byler disease, named after the Amish descendants of Jacob Byler. Clinically, patients present with cholestatic jaundice, pruritus, chronic watery diarrhea, and a failure to thrive as early as the first month of life. In addition to liver involvement, patients also may have pancreatitis, hearing loss, and pneumonia. Despite other features of cholestasis, biochemical tests show normal or low GGT and elevated ALT. Bile acids are elevated in the serum but low in the bile. Because FIC1 protein expression is higher in the intestine than the liver, defects in intestinal absorption may be involved in the pathogenesis of the diarrhea. Treatment is biliary diversion and is most successful if performed before cirrhosis develops.

Histologic Findings

The characteristic histologic finding early in the disease is canalicular cholestasis (bile thrombi). The bile in FIC1 deficiency has a paler color compared with other cholestatic diseases. The lobular architecture is preserved, usually with orderly arranged small hepatocytes (**Fig. 7**A, B).

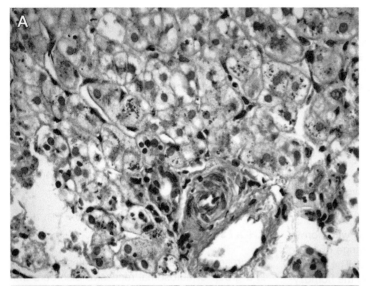

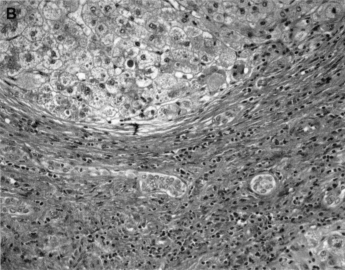

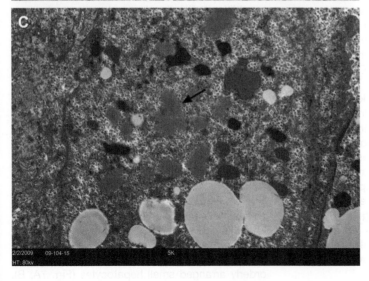

Fig. 6. (*A*) AIAT deficiency, patient with PiZZ phenotype. Periportal granular and globular inclusions in hepatocytes that are PAS-D resistant. The portal tract has absent bile duct. (PAS-D stain, 200×). (*B*) Example of a 6-year-old patient with A1AT deficiency with cirrhosis. Note the hyaline globules at the periphery of the cirrhotic nodule (H&E 100×). (*C*) Electron microscopy showing electron-dense particles of variable size and shape, enclosed by membranes in the endoplasmic reticulum (*arrows*), × 9.000.

Table 3
Distinctive genetic, clinical, and histopathology features of PFICs 1,2,3

	FIC 1 Deficiency (PFIC1)	BSEP Deficiency (PFIC2)	MDR3 Deficiency (PFIC3)
Genetic locus	18q21-22	2q24	7q21
Gene	ATP8B1	ABCB11	ABCB4
Clinical features	Jaundice, severe pruritus, Diarrhea/steatorrhea, growth failure, pancreatitis, deafness, chronic respiratory disease	Jaundice, pruritus, failure to thrive No extrahepatic manifestations	Jaundice, pale stools, pruritus
GGT	Low/Normal	Low/Normal	High
Histologic findings			
Portal	Small interlobular bile ducts	Paucity and ductular reaction, occasionally	Ductular reaction, cholesterol clefts in bile ducts, GCT, focally, rare
Lobular	Preserved architecture Bile thrombi with pale bile; no inflammation	Florid GCT with disarray of lobular architecture	Cholestasis with pseudorosettes
Fibrosis	Portal to portal and centrilobular with slow progression to cirrhosis	Portal to portal with rapid progression to cirrhosis	Biliary cirrhosis with biliary "halo" in periphery of cirrhotic nodules
IHC	No specific IHC antibody	BSEP expression absent in most	MDR3 expression absent in subset
Electron microscopy	Coarse (Byler) bile	Amorphous/finely filamentous	Cholesterol crystal
Hepatobiliary malignancy	Not described	Yes	Yes
Allograft disease	Steatohepatitis	Recurrence of disease	Not known

Abbreviations: BSEP, bile salt export pump; GCT, giant cell transformation; IHC, Immunohistochemistry; PFIC, Progressive familial intrahepatic cholestasis.

Giant cell transformation when present tends to be mild. Later in the disease, bile ductular proliferation and portal and centrilobular fibrosis may supervene. Paucity of interlobular bile ducts has been described. Progressive fibrosis can lead to cirrhosis as early as the second or third year of life and often by the first decade. Electron microscopy shows "Byler bile," which is coarse and granular and is quite distinct from other cholestatic diseases (see **Fig. 7**C). Byler bile is seen in specimens primarily fixed with glutaraldehyde, and not in formalin-fixed tissues.[24]

BSEP DEFICIENCY (FORMERLY PFIC TYPE 2)

BSEP deficiency is caused by mutations of the *ABCB11* gene that encodes a transporter of bile acid located in the canalicular membrane known as bile salt export pump (BSEP). The clinical presentation usually is in the neonatal period with cholestatic jaundice and pruritus. Like FIC1 deficiency, the patient's GGT is normal or low, despite cholestasis. There are, however, markedly elevated aminotransferases. Also unlike FIC1 deficiency, there is no extrahepatic or multiorgan involvement.

Histologic Findings

Liver histologic findings vary with progression of the disease. In infants, disarray of lobular architecture with giant cell transformation of hepatocytes and hepatocellular and canalicular cholestasis are the most common features (**Fig. 8**). Ductular reaction is rarely present but may become more prominent later in the course of the disease. Occasionally, bile duct paucity may develop. The fibrosis begins in the pericentral region. Cirrhosis may develop as early as age 1 year.

Immunohistochemistry is of diagnostic value only when BSEP expression is completely lost. The expression of this marker, however, may vary depending on the type of mutation involved. The diagnosis is best established by molecular testing for the genetic mutation. Both hepatocellular

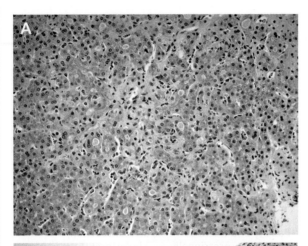

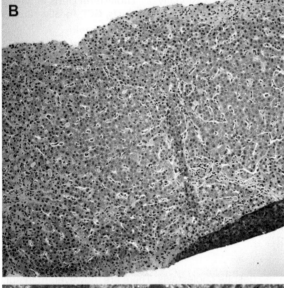

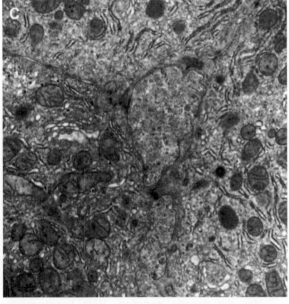

Fig. 7. (*A*) FIC1 deficiency (PFIC1), showing "bile thrombi," with pale bile, which correspond to the coarse granular bile seen by elecron microscopy. Note the portal tracts lack any inflammation or ductular proliferation. (*B*) FIC1 deficiency, cords of small hepatocytes typically seen in this disease. (*C*) Coarse, granular bile, or Byler bile–specific electron microscopy finding in this disease.

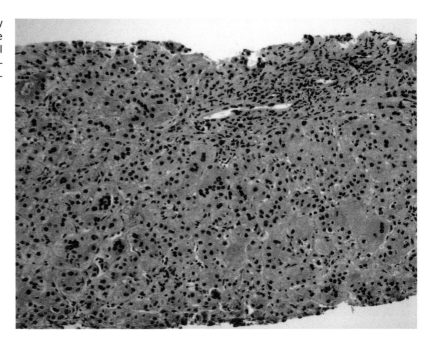

Fig. 8. BSEP deficiency (PFIC2), showing lobule with diffuse giant cell transformation of hepatocytes, canalicular and hepatocellular cholestasis.

carcinoma and cholangiocarcinoma are reported complications of the disease.[25,26]

Treatment of BSEP deficiency is supportive. Partial external biliary diversion has been successful in some patients. Liver transplantation is required in many cases and disease recurrence in the graft is a known complication.[27]

MDR3 DEFICIENCY (FORMERLY PFIC TYPE 3)

MDR3 deficiency is caused by mutations of the *ABCB4* gene that encodes the multidrug-resistant P-glycoprotein, a translocator of phospholipid across the canalicular membrane. Bile with low phospholipids is toxic, leading to biliary disease and propensity to develop gallstones. The clinical presentation with jaundice and acholic stool occurs as early as the first month of life, but more commonly in the first year of life or in young adults. MDR3 deficiency has been associated with various cholestatic disorders in adults, including cholestasis of pregnancy and drug-related cholestasis. In contrast to the 2 other forms of PFICs discussed previously, MDR3 is associated with elevated serum GGT.

Histologic Findings

Ductular proliferation/reaction and portal fibrosis is characteristic, similar to that seen in biliary atresia. Cholestasis is most frequently hepatocellular but canalicular and ductular cholestasis can also be seen. Depending on the nature of mutation and clinical presentation, liver biopsy findings vary. In children, the typical finding is bile ductular proliferation without duct epithelial injury or periductular fibrosis. Interlobular bile ducts are preserved and may contain bile plugs. Lobular and portal inflammatory infiltrate can be seen (**Fig. 9**). Cholesterol clefts can be rarely seen in bile duct lumen, probably reflecting reduced cholesterol solubility. Progression to cirrhosis can manifest as early as 5 months of age.[28] Not all children with the *ABCB4* mutation develop cirrhosis, but approximately 50% of patients develop cirrhosis and progress to liver failure before adolescence. The cirrhosis is of the biliary type with preservation of bile ducts. The differential diagnosis is usually primary sclerosing cholangitis.

Immunostain for MDR3, which normally shows strong canalicular positivity in hepatocytes may be diagnostic in cases when there is complete lack of staining for the protein.[29] A recent study in children with the *ABC4* mutation showed absence or faint staining in hepatocytes (fewer than 5% of cells) in most children carrying the disease-causing mutation on both alleles.[29] A variable reduction of staining (between 20% and 60% of cells) was detected in patients with a mild genotype.[29]

Hepatocellular carcinoma and cholangiocarcinoma have been recently described in patients with MDR3 deficiency.[30]

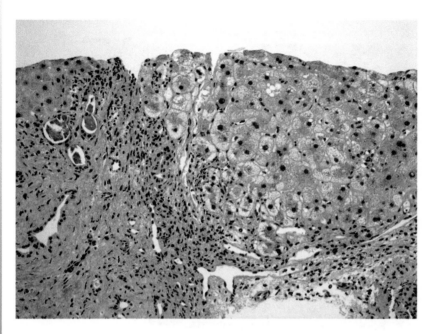

Fig. 9. MDR3 deficiency (PFIC3), in a 17-year-old who presented with cryptogenic cirrhosis. The hepatocytes on the periphery of the cirrhotic nodule show cholate stasis and occasional Mallory hyaline. The fibrotic band has ductular proliferation and prominent ductal cholestasis. This finding can be very focal.

BILE ACID SYNTHETIC DISORDERS

Bile acid synthetic disorders (BASDs) are inborn errors of bile acid synthesis, inherited as an autosomal recessive trait that can produce life-threatening cholestatic liver disease, usually presenting in infancy, and progressive neurologic disease, presenting later in childhood or in adult life. Nine BASDs have been characterized. The enzyme defect, associated genes, and clinical features have been summarized by Sundaram and colleagues.[31] These, along with the main histologic findings, are shown in **Table 4**.

Clinically, BASDs often present in the first few months of life with conjugated hyperbilirubinemia, raised transaminases, and usually normal GGT. Pruritus is usually absent in children with BASD, with the reported exception of children with 3β-HSD. Frequently, there is evidence of fat-soluble vitamin malabsorption. Serum concentrations of the primary bile acids are typically normal or low in affected patients. Hepatobiliary injury is caused by the hepatotoxicity of intermediate metabolites and the absence of the normal trophic and choleretic primary bile acids. Exogenous administration of bile acid can supply adequate luminal concentrations of bile acids and also inhibit the formation of toxic intermediate metabolites. Early recognition allows

institution of targeted bile acid replacement, which reverses the hepatic injury.

Diagnosis is established by fast atom bombardment–mass spectrometry (FAB-MS) and gas chromatography–mass spectrometry of urine and serum, or by sequencing genomic DNA for the specific mutation.

HISTOLOGIC FINDINGS

The histopathological features of BASD overlap with numerous other entities presenting with cholestatic jaundice in childhood. The histologic features most suggestive of BASD include giant cell transformation of hepatocytes with persistence of giant cells in older children. In addition, portal inflammation, necrotic hepatocytes, necrotic giant cells, and ductular proliferation with bile plugs can also be seen. The pathologic findings can be focal and variable.[32,33] In nontreated cases, rapid progression to cirrhosis can be seen. In contrast to other BASDs, Zellweger syndrome and 5βRD show increased iron in hepatocytes. Electron microscopy shows characteristic lack of peroxisomes in Zellweger syndrome.

The most commonly reported BASD defect is 3β-HSD. Histologically, liver biopsy shows disarray of lobular architecture with giant cell formation and necrosis. In addition, portal-to-portal

Table 4
Bile acid synthetic disorders, gene mutation, clinical features, and liver findings

Enzyme Defect	Gene Encoding the Affected Enzyme	Clinical Features	Liver Disease
Oxysterol 7α-hydroxylase deficiency	CYP7 B	Neonatal hepatitis (single reported case; unrecognized cases could be due to prenatal or early-postnatal death)	GCT, lobular disarray, portal tract inflammation and fibrosis, rapid progression to cirrhosis
Δ⁴-3-oxosteroid-5β-reductase deficiency	AKR1D1 (SRD5B1)	Neonatal hepatitis with rapid progression to liver failure Neonatal hemochromatosis	GCT, necrotic hepatocytes. Minimal ductular reaction. Portal and lobular fibrosis. Iron deposition and extensive hepatic necrosis
3β-hydroxy-Δ⁵-C₂₇″ steroid dehydrogenase deficiency	HSD3B7	Neonatal hepatitis Late-onset liver disease Malabsorption	GCT, disarray of lobular architecture, necrosis. Portal-to-portal fibrosis
Cerebrotendinous xanthomatosis (sterol 27-hydroxylase deficiency)	CYP27A1	Progressive neurologic dysfunction in 2nd–3rd decade of life Chronic diarrhea Bilateral juvenile cataracts Neonatal cholestasis	Neonatal hepatitis with GCT, self-limiting, after latent period neurodegenerative disorder ensues
Alpha methylacyl-CoA racemase deficiency	AMACR gene on chromosome 5p13.2-q11.1	Adult-onset peripheral neuropathy Neonatal cholestasis with considerable fat-soluble-vitamin deficiency	GCT, portal inflammation, necrotic hepatocytes, iron storage, reduced peroxisomes
Zellweger syndrome (cerebrohepatorenal syndrome)	12 PEX gene mutations; PEX1 mutations are the most common	Craniofacial abnormalities Neuronal migration defects Polycystic kidneys Chronic liver disease Bony abnormalities	Mild inflammation Bile ductular proliferation Septal and lobular fibrosis Paucity of bile ducts Iron deposition Absence of peroxisomes
Bile acid conjugation defects	BAAT and BAL	Transient neonatal cholestasis Fat-soluble vitamin deficiencies	Transient or no liver disease

Abbreviation: GCT, giant cell transformation.

bridging fibrosis and portal and lobular inflammation are often present. Bile duct proliferation is generally lacking in these cases.[34]

DIFFERENTIAL DIAGNOSIS

Depending on the histology, bile salt transporter defects, idiopathic giant cell (neonatal) hepatitis, biliary atresia, and neonatal iron storage disease need to be considered in the differential diagnosis.

GIANT CELL HEPATITIS (NEONATAL GIANT CELL HEPATITIS, IDIOPATHIC NEONATAL HEPATITIS, IDIOPATHIC NEONATAL GIANT CELL HEPATITIS)

Idiopathic neonatal giant cell hepatitis (NGCH) currently is a diagnosis of exclusion, as many such cases diagnosed in the past are now recognized as other bile salt transport defects (familial

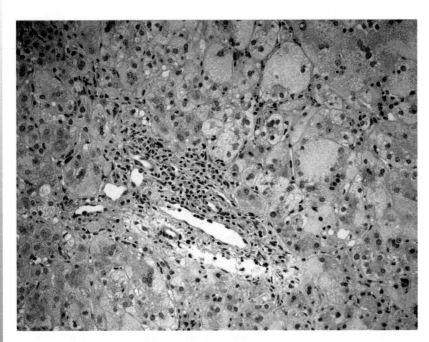

Fig. 10. Neonatal giant cell hepatitis (GCH) showing prominent giant cell transformation and portal tract with no visible bile ducts.

intrahepatic cholestasis syndromes), BASD, and others. Giant cell transformation of hepatocytes is a nonspecific finding and is probably a reactive change very commonly seen in a variety of cholestatic diseases of children.

HISTOLOGIC FINDINGS

Histologically NGCH is characterized by the formation of syncytial hepatic giant cells, variable inflammation, and predominantly lobular or canalicular cholestasis. Duct or ductular proliferation, or paucity of bile duct is not a feature, and should suggest an alternative diagnosis. A subset (up to 16%) of NGCH has been related to hypopituitarism and these cases have hypoplastic bile ducts (**Fig. 10**), which without the aid of keratin stain, could be easily overlooked.[35]

Autoimmune hemolytic anemia with giant cell hepatitis (GCH) is an uncommon disease in children and is often associated with a fatal course. It is suggested that GCH in combination with hemolytic anemia is a unique autoimmune disorder. Liver failure is the leading cause of death in these children. Response to prednisone and rituximab has been reported.[36]

REFERENCES

1. Moyer V, Freese DK, Whitington PF, et al. Guideline for the evaluation of cholestatic jaundice in infants: recommendations of the North American Society for Pediatric Gastroenterology, Hepatology and Nutrition. J Pediatr Gastroenterol Nutr 2004;39(2): 115–28.
2. Balistreri WF, Bezerra JA. Whatever happened to "neonatal hepatitis"? Clin Liver Dis 2006;10(1): 27–53, v.
3. Sokol RJ, Shepherd RW, Superina R, et al. Screening and outcomes in biliary atresia: summary of a National Institutes of Health workshop. Hepatology 2007;46(2):566–81.
4. Davenport M, Tizzard SA, Underhill J, et al. The biliary atresia splenic malformation syndrome: a 28-year single-center retrospective study. J Pediatr 2006;149(3):393–400.
5. Chardot C, Serinet MO. Prognosis of biliary atresia: what can be further improved? J Pediatr 2006; 148(4):432–5.
6. Weerasooriya VS, White FV, Shepherd RW. Hepatic fibrosis and survival in biliary atresia. J Pediatr 2004;144(1):123–5.
7. Russo P, Magee JC, Boitnott J, et al. Design and validation of the biliary atresia research consortium histologic assessment system for cholestasis in infancy. Clin Gastroenterol Hepatol 2011;9(4):357–362.e2.
8. Brough AJ, Bernstein J. Conjugated hyperbilirubinemia in early infancy. A reassessment of liver biopsy. Hum Pathol 1974;5(5):507–16.
9. Manolaki AG, Larcher VF, Mowat AP, et al. The prelaparotomy diagnosis of extrahepatic biliary atresia. Arch Dis Child 1983;58(8):591–4.

10. Rastogi A, Krishnani N, Yachha SK, et al. Histopathological features and accuracy for diagnosing biliary atresia by prelaparotomy liver biopsy in developing countries. J Gastroenterol Hepatol 2009;24(1): 97–102.

11. Brunati A, Feruzi Z, Sokal E, et al. Early occurrence of hepatocellular carcinoma in biliary atresia treated by liver transplantation. Pediatr Transplant 2007; 11(1):117–9.

12. Fitzgibbons SC, Jones BA, Hull MA, et al. Relationship between biopsy-proven parenteral nutrition-associated liver fibrosis and biochemical cholestasis in children with short bowel syndrome. J Pediatr Surg 2010;45(1):95–9 [discussion: 99].

13. Zambrano E, El-Hennawy M, Ehrenkranz RA, et al. Total parenteral nutrition induced liver pathology: an autopsy series of 24 newborn cases. Pediatr Dev Pathol 2004;7(5):425–32.

14. Naini BV, Lassman CR. Total parenteral nutrition therapy and liver injury: a histopathologic study with clinical correlation. Hum Pathol 2012;43(6):826–33.

15. Patterson K, Kapur SP, Chandra RS. Hepatocellular carcinoma in a noncirrhotic infant after prolonged parenteral nutrition. J Pediatr 1985;106(5):797–800.

16. Girard M, Franchi-Abella S, Lacaille F, et al. Specificities of sclerosing cholangitis in childhood. Clin Res Hepatol Gastroenterol 2012;36(6):530–5.

17. Miloh T, Arnon R, Shneider B, et al. A retrospective single-center review of primary sclerosing cholangitis in children. Clin Gastroenterol Hepatol 2009;7(2): 239–45.

18. Hadchouel M. Paucity of interlobular bile ducts. Semin Diagn Pathol 1992;9(1):24–30.

19. Markowitz J, Daum F, Kahn EI, et al. Arteriohepatic dysplasia. I. Pitfalls in diagnosis and management. Hepatology 1983;3(1):74–6.

20. Subramaniam P, Knisely A, Portmann B, et al. Diagnosis of Alagille syndrome—25 years of experience at King's College Hospital. J Pediatr Gastroenterol Nutr 2011;52(1):84–9.

21. Bhadri VA, Stormon MO, Arbuckle S, et al. Hepatocellular carcinoma in children with Alagille syndrome. J Pediatr Gastroenterol Nutr 2005;41(5):676–8.

22. Rudnick DA, Perlmutter DH. Alpha-1-antitrypsin deficiency: a new paradigm for hepatocellular carcinoma in genetic liver disease. Hepatology 2005; 42(3):514–21.

23. Zhou H, Fischer HP. Liver carcinoma in PiZ alpha-1-antitrypsin deficiency. Am J Surg Pathol 1998;22(6): 742–8.

24. Bull LN, Carlton VE, Stricker NL, et al. Genetic and morphological findings in progressive familial intrahepatic cholestasis (Byler disease [PFIC-1] and Byler syndrome): evidence for heterogeneity. Hepatology 1997;26(1):155–64.

25. Scheimann AO, Strautnieks SS, Knisely AS, et al. Mutations in bile salt export pump (ABCB11) in two children with progressive familial intrahepatic cholestasis and cholangiocarcinoma. J Pediatr 2007;150(5):556–9.

26. Knisely AS, Strautnieks SS, Meier Y, et al. Hepatocellular carcinoma in ten children under five years of age with bile salt export pump deficiency. Hepatology 2006;44(2):478–86.

27. Jara P, Hierro L, Martinez-Fernandez P, et al. Recurrence of bile salt export pump deficiency after liver transplantation. N Engl J Med 2009;361(14): 1359–67.

28. Jacquemin E, De Vree JM, Cresteil D, et al. The wide spectrum of multidrug resistance 3 deficiency: from neonatal cholestasis to cirrhosis of adulthood. Gastroenterology 2001;120(6):1448–58.

29. Colombo C, Vajro P, Degiorgio D, et al. Clinical features and genotype-phenotype correlations in children with progressive familial intrahepatic cholestasis type 3 related to ABCB4 mutations. J Pediatr Gastroenterol Nutr 2011;52(1):73–83.

30. Wendum D, Barbu V, Rosmorduc O, et al. Aspects of liver pathology in adult patients with MDR3/ABCB4 gene mutations. Virchows Arch 2012;460(3): 291–8.

31. Sundaram SS, Bove KE, Lovell MA, et al. Mechanisms of disease: inborn errors of bile acid synthesis. Nat Clin Pract Gastroenterol Hepatol 2008;5(8): 456–68.

32. Bove KE, Daugherty CC, Tyson W, et al. Bile acid synthetic defects and liver disease. Pediatr Dev Pathol 2000;3(1):1–16.

33. Bove KE, Heubi JE, Balistreri WF, et al. Bile acid synthetic defects and liver disease: a comprehensive review. Pediatr Dev Pathol 2004;7(4):315–34.

34. Subramaniam P, Clayton PT, Portmann BC, et al. Variable clinical spectrum of the most common inborn error of bile acid metabolism—3beta-hydroxy-Delta 5-C27-steroid dehydrogenase deficiency. J Pediatr Gastroenterol Nutr 2010;50(1):61–6.

35. Torbenson M, Hart J, Westerhoff M, et al. Neonatal giant cell hepatitis: histological and etiological findings. Am J Surg Pathol 2010;34(10): 1498–503.

36. Miloh T, Manwani D, Morotti R, et al. Giant cell hepatitis and autoimmune hemolytic anemia successfully treated with rituximab. J Pediatr Gastroenterol Nutr 2007;44(5):634–6.

Nonalcoholic Steatohepatitis
Diagnostic Challenges

Ryan M. Gill, MD, PhD*, Sanjay Kakar, MD

KEYWORDS

• Pathology • Steatohepatitis • Diagnosis • Fatty liver disease • NASH

ABSTRACT

This article reviews diagnostic criteria for nonalcoholic steatohepatitis (NASH), current grading and staging methodology, and diagnostic challenges and pitfalls in routine practice. Current practice guidelines and prognostic and treatment considerations are discussed. The clinical diagnosis of nonalcoholic fatty liver disease may represent stable disease without progressive liver damage, in the form of nonalcoholic fatty liver (NAFL), or aggressive disease that will progress to advanced fibrosis, in the form of NASH. NASH is diagnosed from a liver biopsy after assessment by a pathologist to distinguish NASH from NAFL (and other histologic mimics of NASH); this distinction is critical for patient management.

OVERVIEW

Nonalcoholic fatty liver disease (NAFLD) indicates evidence of fat in the liver, either by imaging or histology, in a patient without a reason to have secondary fat accumulation (eg, significant alcohol consumption, use of certain medications, or inherited storage defects; Table 1). Significant alcohol consumption for the purpose of clinical consideration of fatty liver is defined as ongoing or recent consumption of more than 21 drinks on average per week for men, and more than 14 drinks on average per week for women.[1]

Histologic examination of liver tissue is required to subclassify NAFLD as nonalcoholic fatty liver (NAFL) or nonalcoholic steatohepatitis (NASH).[1] NAFL represents steatosis without histologic liver injury, whereas NASH represents steatosis with histologic evidence of liver injury (ie, ballooned hepatocytes, inflammation, and fibrosis, see *Key features box*). The risk of progression to advanced fibrosis in NAFL is minimal whereas in NASH, progression to cirrhosis and/or development of hepatocellular carcinoma (HCC) is well described.[2] NASH cirrhosis is defined as cirrhosis with current or previous evidence of NAFLD.

The median worldwide prevalence of NAFLD is estimated at 20% and the prevalence of NASH reportedly ranges between 3% and 5%.[1,2] The prevalence of NAFLD in the overweight/obese US adult population is probably significantly higher.[1] Risk factors for NASH include metabolic syndrome, dyslipidemia, diabetes mellitus type 2, and obesity (Table 2).[1] Metabolic syndrome is defined as central obesity and insulin resistance, which characteristically manifests with at least 3 of the following:

1. Blood pressure greater than 130/85 mm Hg
2. Increased waist circumference (greater than 102 cm in men and greater than 88 cm in women)
3. Fasting blood sugar level greater than 110 mg/dL
4. Triglycerides greater than 150 mg/dL
5. Low high-density lipoprotein level (<40 mg/dL in men, <50 mg/dL in women)

> ### Key Pathologic Features
> ### NASH
>
> • Steatosis greater than 5%
>
> • Mixed acinar inflammation
>
> • Hepatocellular ballooning and/or pericellular fibrosis

Department of Pathology, University of California, San Francisco, 505 Parnassus Avenue, M590, Box 0102, San Francisco, CA 94143-0102, USA
* Corresponding author.
E-mail address: ryan.gill@ucsf.edu

Surgical Pathology 6 (2013) 227–257
http://dx.doi.org/10.1016/j.path.2013.03.002
1875-9181/13/$ – see front matter © 2013 Elsevier Inc. All rights reserved.

Table 1
Secondary hepatic macrovesicular fat deposition

Excess alcohol	Abetalipoproteinemia
Hepatitis C (particularly genotype 3)	Medications (eg)
Wilson disease	Amiodarone
Lipodystrophy	Methotrexate
Starvation	Tamoxifen
Parenteral nutrition	Corticosteroids

Table 2
Risk factors for NASH

Metabolic diseases (acquired)	Drugs
	Definite association
Obesity	Amiodarone
Diabetes, type 2	Chemotherapeutic
Hypertriglyceridemia	agents (eg
Rapid weight loss	irinotecan)
Malnutrition	Questionable
Metabolic diseases (genetic)	association;
	Tamoxifen
Wilson disease	Steroids
Tyrosinemia	Estrogens
Abetalipoproteinemia	Diethylstilbestrol
Other	Methotrexate
Lipodystrophy	Calcium channel
Jejunoileal bypass	blockers (eg nifedipine, verapamil, and diltiazem)

There are no clinical or radiologic tests that can reliably diagnose steatohepatitis and serum transaminases often correlate poorly with biopsy findings.[1,3] Microscopic examination of a liver biopsy by a pathologist remains the gold standard for diagnosis of NAFLD.

Comprehensive practice guidelines have recently been published for the diagnosis and management of NAFLD[1]; some of these recommendations (Chalasani and colleagues[1] make a total of 45 recommendations) are highlighted in this review. For example, it is recommended that liver biopsy should be considered in all patients with NAFLD who are at increased risk for steatohepatitis and advanced fibrosis. They recommend that the presence of metabolic syndrome and the NAFLD fibrosis score be used to identify patients who are at increased risk for steatohepatitis and advanced fibrosis.[1] Liver biopsy should also be considered in patients with NAFLD if there are competing causes

for hepatic steatosis (as detected by imaging) and whenever coexisting chronic liver disease cannot be excluded without a liver biopsy.[1] Biopsy is currently not recommended in asymptomatic patients with incidental hepatic steatosis on imaging and no other evidence of liver disease.[1]

MICROSCOPIC FEATURES

Three microscopic features are essential for the diagnosis of steatohepatitis (**Table 3**)[4,5]: steatosis, inflammation, and hepatocellular injury in the form

Table 3
Histologic features of nonalcoholic steatohepatitis

Essential features	Often present, not essential for diagnosis
1. Steatosis, predominantly macrovesicular, concentrated in zone 3	1. Glycogenated nuclei in zone 1
2. Mild mixed acinar inflammation	2. Lipogranulomas in the lobular parenchyma or portal tracts
3. Hepatocellular injury in the form of	3. Occasional acidophil bodies
a. Hepatocellular ballooning, often most prominent in zone 3, and/or	
b. Pericellular fibrosis	
May be present, not essential for diagnosis	**Unusual features**
1. Mallory hyaline in zone 3, typically inconspicuous	1. Predominantly microvesicular steatosis
2. Mild iron deposits in hepatocytes or sinusoidal cells	2. Prominent portal and/or acinar inflammation, numerous plasma cells
3. Megamitochondria	3. Prominent bile ductular reaction, cholestasis
	4. Perivenular fibrosis, hyaline sclerosis
	5. Marked lobular inflammation

Adapted from the American Association for the Study of Liver Diseases (AASLD) conference summary on NASH, 2002; and Data from Neuschwander-Tetri BA, Caldwell SH. Nonalcoholic steatohepatitis: summary of an AASLD Single Topic Conference. Hepatology 2003;37(5):1202–19.

Fig. 1. Mild steatosis, 5% to 32%, macrovesicular (large and small droplet), hematoxylin and eosin (H&E) stain, magnification ×100.

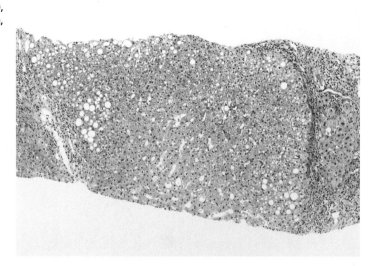

of hepatocyte ballooning and/or pericentral fibrosis. Significant steatosis is defined as greater than 5% macrovesicular steatosis (includes both large-droplet and small-droplet fat), usually with pericentral accentuation (Figs. 1–3). Inflammation is usually mild and more prominent in the lobular parenchyma (Fig. 4), with or without a component of mild portal inflammation (Fig. 5). Neutrophils are typically present, usually in small numbers, but can surround ballooned hepatocytes (ie, neutrophil satellitosis) (Fig. 6), as is more commonly seen in alcoholic steatohepatitis. Lymphocytes and histiocytes are also common with lipogranuloma formation (Fig. 7) often noted. Occasional eosinophils, pigmented macrophages, and microgranulomas

may be present. Steatohepatitic hepatocellular injury manifests as ballooned hepatocytes or, in the chronic phase, as pericellular fibrosis around central veins. Hepatocellular ballooning is characterized by an increase in cell size, rarefaction of cytoplasm, and condensation of cytoplasm into eosinophilic globular areas (Figs. 8 and 9).[4] When conspicuous, the globular structures are referred to as Mallory hyaline (Fig. 10). All 3 characteristics must be present for definite interpretation as hepatocellular ballooning. Hepatocytes with small-droplet steatosis (Fig. 11) or with excessive glycogen (Fig. 12) can be enlarged or clear, but do not have all 3 characteristics and should not be interpreted as ballooned

Fig. 2. Moderate steatosis, 33% to 65%, macrovesicular (large and small droplet), H&E stain, magnification ×100.

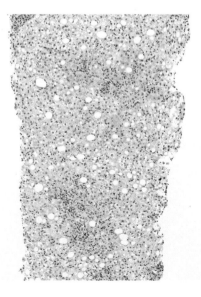

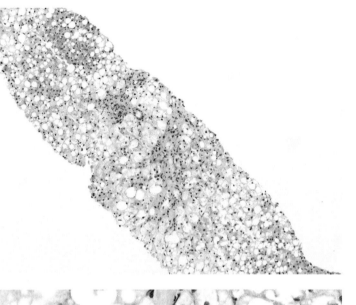

Fig. 3. Severe steatosis, 66% to 100%, mostly macrovesicular (large and small droplet), H&E stain, magnification ×100.

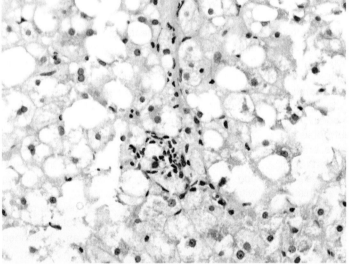

Fig. 4. A focus of lobular inflammation in steatohepatitis, H&E stain, magnification ×400.

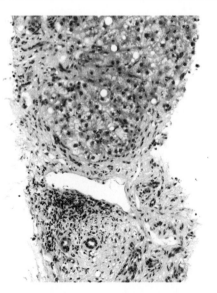

Fig. 5. One portal tract with mild portal inflammation in a case of steatohepatitis, H&E stain, magnification ×200.

Fig. 6. Focal neutrophil satellitosis in a case of steatohepatitis, H&E stain, magnification ×400.

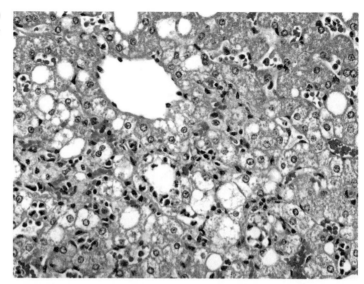

Fig. 7. Lipogranuloma formation in the lobular parenchyma in a case of steatohepatitis (*arrow*), H&E stain, magnification ×400.

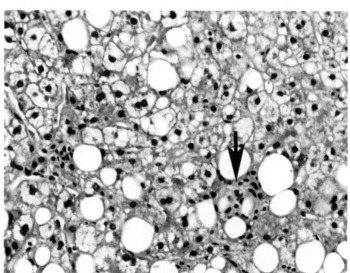

Fig. 8. Pericentral ballooned hepatocytes (*arrow*) in a case of steatohepatitis, H&E stain, magnification ×200.

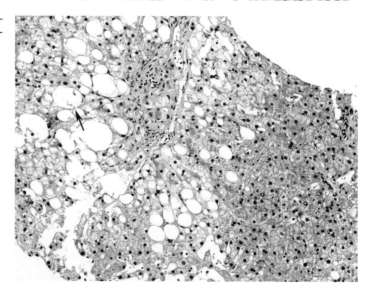

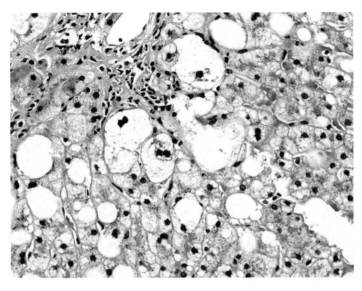

Fig. 9. Multiple ballooned hepato-cytes in a case of steatohepatitis, H&E stain, magnification ×400.

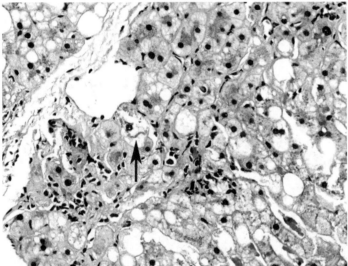

Fig. 10. Mallory hyaline (arrow) in ballooned hepatocytes in a case of steatohepatitis, H&E stain, magnification ×400.

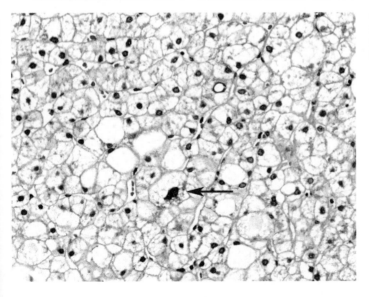

Fig. 11. Ballooned hepatocyte mimic (arrow) with small-droplet fat in a case of severe steatosis without fibrosis, H&E stain, magnification ×400.

Fig. 12. Ballooned hepatocyte mimic (*arrow*) with glycogenated cytoplasm in a case of mild steatosis without fibrosis, H&E stain, magnification ×400.

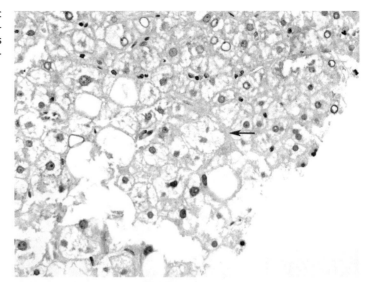

Fig. 13. Spotty hepatocyte necrosis (*arrowheads*), some with intracellular fat, in a case of steatohepatitis, H&E stain, magnification ×400.

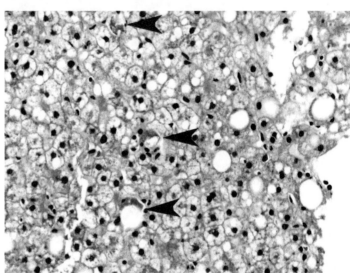

Fig. 14. Pericentral/sinusoidal fibrosis in steatohepatitis, stage 1 (Brunt methodology, scale 0–4), trichrome stain, magnification ×200.

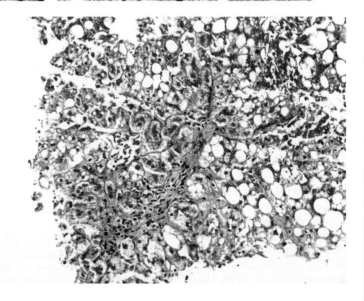

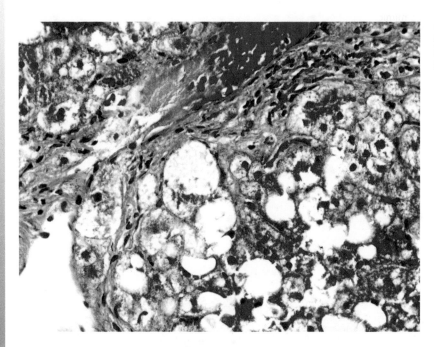

Fig. 15. Pericentral/sinu-soidal fibrosis in steato-hepatitis, trichrome stain, magnification ×400.

hepatocytes. Spotty hepatocyte necrosis (**Fig. 13**) is also common and does not necessarily support a viral etiology. Pericellular fibrosis involving sinu-soids in zone 3 results in a chicken-wire or spider-web pattern of fibrosis (**Figs. 14** and **15**).

NASH GRADING AND STAGING

The extent of fibrosis documented in a biopsy can influence clinical decisions and should always be included in the pathology report as the fibrosis stage. For example, the presence of fibrosis may prompt the hepatologist to pursue underlying risk factors more aggressively and treatment con-siderations may include more aggressive manage-ment (eg, gastric bypass surgery for obesity or enrollment in clinical trials). The degree of fibrosis is important for monitoring disease progression in subsequent biopsies and documentation of ad-vanced fibrosis (stage 3 or 4) allows for adequate planning for transplantation. Unlike chronic viral hepatitis, which is a portal-based disease, fibrosis in steatohepatitis typically starts around the cen-tral vein. Therefore, the staging systems used in chronic viral hepatitis, such as the Batts-Ludwig methodology,[6] are not appropriate for NASH. Two staging schemas are available for NASH, the Brunt methodology[7] and the NASH clinical research network (CRN)/Kleiner[5] modification to

this methodology (**Tables 4** and **5**). In practice, the Brunt methodology is sufficient for most clin-ical reports (see **Figs. 14** and **15**; **Figs. 16–18**).

In addition to the general pitfalls of staging chronic hepatitis (eg, subcapsular biopsy, frag-mentation, limited sample, tangentially cut portal tracts) (**Fig. 19**), some problems specific to steato-hepatitis include trichrome staining quality (over-staining can lead to a trichrome stain with thin

Table 4		
Staging of steatohepatitis: Brunt methodology		
Stage 0	No fibrosis	
Stage 1	Zone 3 pericellular/sinusoidal fibrosis, focal or extensive	
Stage 2	As in stage 1 plus portal fibrosis, focal or extensive	
Stage 3	Bridging fibrosis, focal or extensive	
Stage 4	Cirrhosis (± residual pericellular fibrosis)	

Data from Brunt EM, Janney CG, Di Bisceglie AM, et al. Nonalcoholic steatohepatitis: a proposal for grading and staging the histologic lesions. Am J Gastroenterol 1999; 94(9):2467–74.

Table 5
Staging of steatohepatitis: NASH CRN modified Brunt methodology

Stage 0	No fibrosis

Stage 1	Perisinusoidal or periportal fibrosis
	  1A. Mild zone 3 pericellular fibrosis, requires trichrome for identification
	  1B. Moderate zone 3 pericellular fibrosis, often apparent on H&E stain
	  1C. Portal/periportal fibrosis only

Stage 2	As in stage 1 plus portal/periportal fibrosis, focal or extensive
Stage 3	Bridging fibrosis, focal or extensive
Stage 4	Cirrhosis (± residual pericellular fibrosis)

Data from Kleiner DE, Brunt EM, Van Natta M, et al. Design and validation of a histologic scoring system for nonalcoholic fatty liver disease. Hepatology 2005;41(6): 1313–21.

blue strands lining the sinusoids mimicking pericellular fibrosis) (**Fig. 20**), lipogranuloma-related staining (**Fig. 21**) (ie, focal areas of fibrosis in a nodular configuration, especially around central veins, may be caused by lipogranulomas and should not be considered in staging; fibrosis should be considered to be present only if pericellular extension along the sinusoids is seen), and recognition of portal-based fibrosis in the absence of pericellular fibrosis around the central vein, which although uncommon in steatohepatitis, can occur in children and some adult patients with NASH.[8]

Unlike staging, the clinical usefulness of grading in steatohepatitis is not clearly established. At present, clinical decisions are not dictated by the histologic grade. Therefore, grading of steatohepatitis is not considered a necessary component of the pathology report. Hepatologists are often interested in the grade of steatosis (as described in **Table 6**), but not in grading of other elements such as inflammation and ballooning.

The NAFLD activity score (NAS) scheme[5] builds on the earlier Brunt grading scheme[7] and is used by the NASH CRN in case evaluation (see **Table 6**). The NAS is defined as the sum of the scores for steatosis (0–3), lobular inflammation (0–3), and hepatocellular ballooning (0–2). The NAS can therefore range from 0 to 8. The NAS is not intended to replace a pathologist's diagnostic determination of steatohepatitis, but can be reported if grading is desired.

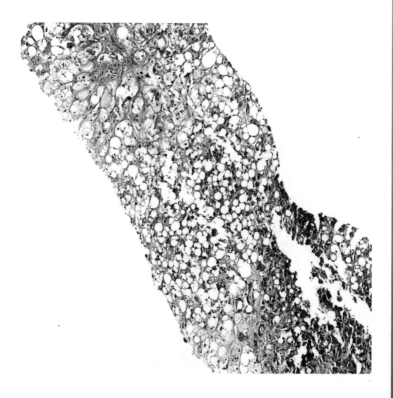

Fig. 16. Steatohepatitis with pericentral and periportal fibrosis, stage 2 (Brunt methodology, scale 0–4), trichrome stain, magnification ×100.

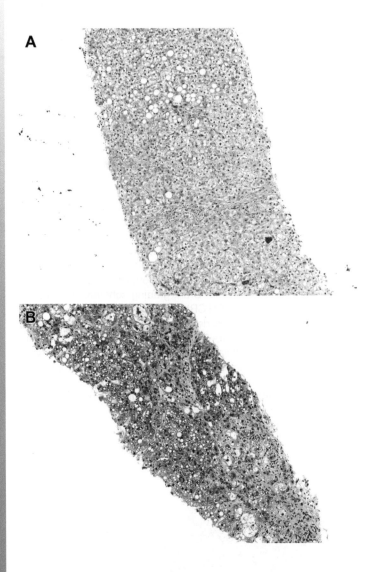

Fig. 17. Steatohepatitis with bridging fibrosis (*A, B*), stage 3 (Brunt methodology, scale 0–4), trichrome stain, magnification ×100.

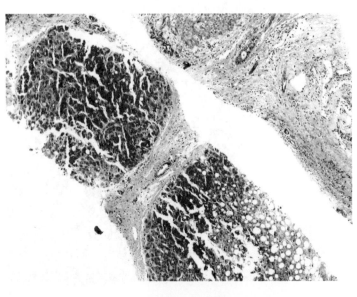

Fig. 18. Steatohepatitis with cirrhosis, stage 4 (Brunt methodology, scale 0–4), trichrome stain, magnification ×100.

Fig. 19. Fibrosis pitfalls; tangentially cut portal tracts (*A, B*) and subcapsular biopsy (*C*), trichrome stains, magnification ×100–200.

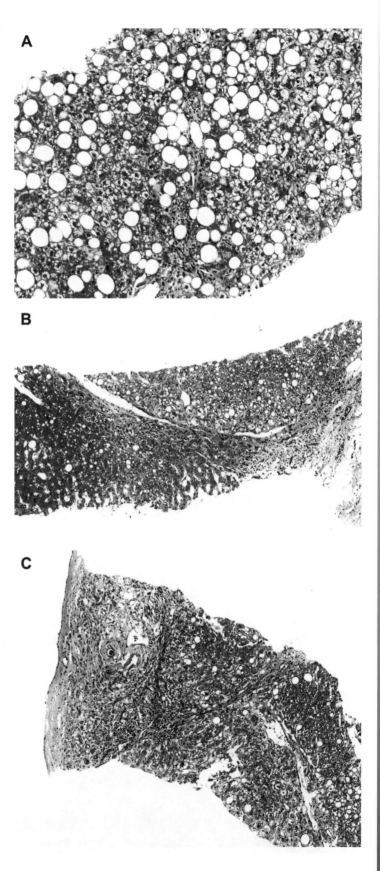

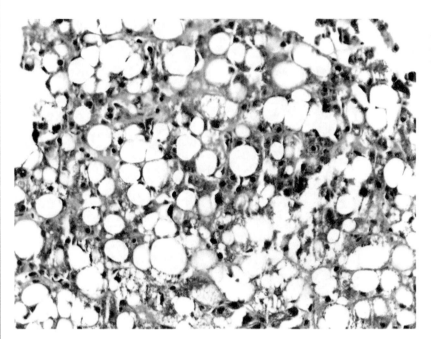

Fig. 20. Overstained trichrome stain mimics pericellular fibrosis, trichrome stain, magnification ×400.

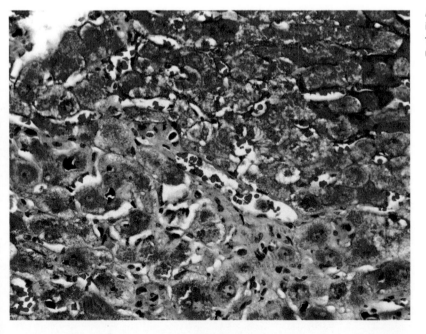

Fig. 21. Kupffer cell staining mimics pericellular fibrosis, trichrome stain, magnification ×400.

Table 6
NASH activity score (NAS)

Histologic Feature	Definition	Score
Steatosis	<5%	0
	5%–33%	1
	>33%–66%	2
	>66%	3
Lobular inflammation[a]	None	0
	<2 foci	1
	2–4 foci	2
	>4 foci	3
Ballooning[b]	None	0
	Few cells	1
	Prominent	2

[a] The number of foci was counted per 200× field for lobular inflammation.
[b] Few ballooned cells indicate rare but definite ballooned hepatocytes as well as cases that are diagnostically borderline.
Data from Kleiner DE, Brunt EM, Van Natta M, et al. Design and validation of a histologic scoring system for nonalcoholic fatty liver disease. Hepatology 2005;41(6): 1313–21.

DIFFERENTIAL DIAGNOSIS

Although many cases of NASH have classic morphologic features of pericentral ballooned hepatocytes, significant steatosis, lobular mixed inflammation, and pericellular fibrosis, we have encountered several variations of these classic features, which can result in diagnostic confusion. Overall, there are 6 patterns of NAFLD to recognize (see *NAFLD patterns of injury box*):

PATTERN 1: STEATOSIS WITH MILD INFLAMMATION, HEPATOCELLULAR BALLOONING, AND/OR PERICELLULAR FIBROSIS

Pattern 1 is a classic steatohepatitis pattern of injury, which can be considered chronic active steatohepatitis.

PATTERN 2: STEATOSIS WITHOUT HEPATOCELLULAR INJURY

Steatosis without hepatocellular injury in the form of ballooning or pericellular fibrosis is insufficient for a diagnosis of steatohepatitis and therefore represents NAFL, which has a low rate of progression (<5%) to significant fibrosis or cirrhosis.[9]

PATTERN 3: STEATOSIS WITH SWOLLEN HEPATOCYTES

Hepatocellular ballooning should be interpreted only if all 3 features of ballooning are present (ie, swelling, cytoplasmic clearing, and condensation of cytoplasm into eosinophilic globular areas). Well-formed Mallory hyaline is not an essential feature, but supports the diagnosis when present. If clear-cut hepatocellular ballooning is not present, but hepatocellular changes are suspicious for ballooning (**Fig. 22**), then the findings should be regarded as borderline for steatohepatitis and it may be best to manage the patient as appropriate for steatohepatitis. It is believed that injured hepatocytes in steatohepatitis have defective protein turnover with ubiquitination and loss of keratin 8/18 (and thus loss of keratin 8/18 by immunohistochemical staining may be used for identification of ballooned hepatocytes in challenging cases).[10,11]

PATTERN 4: BALLOONED HEPATOCYTES OR PERICELLULAR FIBROSIS WITHOUT STEATOSIS

Ballooned hepatocytes without steatosis can be seen with amiodarone use or in patients who have recently stopped taking alcohol. This pattern is uncommon in patients with metabolic risk factors. In addition to steatohepatitis, pericentral/sinusoidal fibrosis can be seen in chronic vascular outflow obstruction or parenchymal rejection (after liver transplant). Sinusoidal fibrosis also occurs in diabetic hepatosclerosis, but tends to be patchy and nonzonal.

⚠️ **Differential Diagnosis**
NAFLD Patterns of Injury[a]

1. Steatosis, mixed inflammation, ballooned hepatocytes, and pericellular fibrosis → NASH

2. Steatosis without hepatocellular injury → NAFL

3. Steatosis with swollen hepatocytes → NAFL versus borderline NASH

4. Ballooned hepatocytes or pericellular fibrosis without steatosis → NASH in the appropriate clinical context

5. Pericellular fibrosis and steatosis, no ballooned hepatocytes → NASH

6. Cirrhosis with steatosis or history of NAFLD risk factors → NASH cirrhosis

[a] Classification as a form of NAFLD requires no history of significant alcohol consumption.

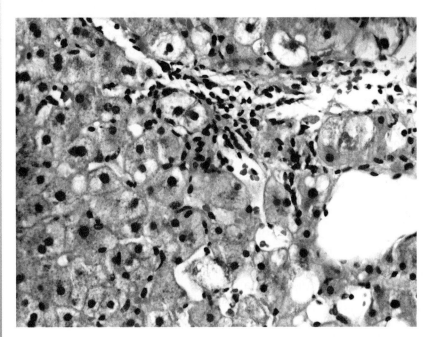

Fig. 22. Hepatocellular changes suspicious for, but not diagnostic of, hepatocellular ballooning (cytoplasmic clearing and globules, but not clearly large enough), H&E stain, magnification ×400.

PATTERN 5: STEATOSIS WITH PERICELLULAR FIBROSIS, BUT NO BALLOONED HEPATOCYTES

In the absence of ballooning, these changes are likely to represent chronic steatohepatitic injury. Pericellular fibrosis can also be a result of chronic venous outflow obstruction (as in right heart failure or Budd-Chiari syndrome), chemotherapeutic agents such as oxaliplatin (a drug used to treat colorectal cancer), or, in the posttransplant setting, with remote parenchymal rejection, as noted for pattern 4, but together with significant steatosis, steatohepatitis is the likely cause. Other possible causes can be mentioned in the pathology report, depending on the clinical context.

PATTERN 6: CIRRHOSIS WITH STEATOSIS AND/OR BALLOONED HEPATOCYTES

Cirrhosis with histologic evidence of NAFLD is best considered NASH cirrhosis (see **Fig. 18**). Some cases may also show residual pericellular fibrosis, although this is somewhat less specific in the setting of established cirrhosis. Over time, the features of NAFLD often disappear (ie, burn out) in cirrhosis, as described later.

DIAGNOSTIC CHALLENGES AND PITFALLS

Beyond the common patterns of NAFLD, many clinical and diagnostic scenarios can present

challenges to the pathologist. The following 9 scenarios are described to assist in avoiding common pitfalls in NASH diagnosis (see *NASH pitfalls box*):

ALCOHOLIC STEATOHEPATITIS

It is usually not possible to definitively distinguish alcoholic from nonalcoholic steatohepatitis based on liver histology. In general, NASH is characterized by more prominent steatosis and less severe

Pitfalls
NASH

! Alcoholic steatohepatitis

! Burnt-out NASH cirrhosis

! Centrizonal arterialization

! Drug-induced liver injury and steatohepatitis

! Hereditary hemochromatosis

! Metabolic disorders (glycogenic hepatopathy, diabetic hepatosclerosis, Wilson disease)

! Microvesicular steatosis

! More than mild portal inflammation

! Pediatric NASH

! Steatohepatitis with an acute/subacute presentation

signs of hepatocellular injury such as ballooning and inflammation. There are also certain histologic features that can occur in alcoholic steatohepatitis, but are less common in NASH, such as abundant Mallory hyaline, prominent neutrophil infiltrate (with neutrophil satellitosis), cholestasis, and obliteration of central veins.

BURNT-OUT NASH CIRRHOSIS

The typical features of steatohepatitis often regress with progression of fibrosis and may be lost with cirrhosis (ie, burnt-out steatohepatitis). These cases end up being labeled as cryptogenic cirrhosis. Because the patient population with cryptogenic cirrhosis has a high prevalence of obesity and type 2 diabetes, it is thought that most cases of cryptogenic cirrhosis are related to nonalcoholic steatohepatitis.[12] In this setting, the correct diagnosis can only be established by ruling out other causes and through correlation with risk factors for steatohepatitis.

CENTRIZONAL ARTERIALIZATION

Identification of arterioles is often helpful in orientation of a liver biopsy, because they normally constitute 1 component of the portal triad. However, arterioles can also be seen in central zones in NASH liver biopsies,[13] most commonly with advanced fibrosis (Fig. 23).[13] This scenario may result in misidentification of a central zone as a portal tract and thereby lead to an erroneous interpretation of a portal-based disease process, potentially resulting in a missed NASH diagnosis.

DRUG-INDUCED LIVER INJURY AND STEATOHEPATITIS

Most cases of NASH can be attributed to obesity, type 2 diabetes, and hyperlipidemia and, among patients with NASH, most have metabolic syndrome. NASH may represent a hepatic component of the metabolic syndrome. However, in patients without risk factors, histologic findings identical to NASH have been observed, so it may not be possible to separate drug-induced steatohepatitis from NASH in some clinical scenarios (see Tables 1 and 2).[14] Amiodarone, irinotecan, perhexiline, and diethylaminoethoxyhexestrol are drugs with a definite association with steatohepatitis.

Amiodarone

Amiodarone, a potent antiarrhythmic agent, causes increased liver enzymes in up to 30% of patients and steatohepatitis in ~1% to 2% of patients.[15–17] Amiodarone steatohepatitis is characterized by prominent Mallory hyaline (occasionally in zone 1) and neutrophil satellitosis, whereas steatosis is less conspicuous (Fig. 24). The findings can be similar to alcoholic steatohepatitis.[15] Reversal of liver injury often occurs with discontinuation of the drug, but may be delayed by weeks or months. In addition, amiodarone is also associated with phospholipidosis, which is characterized

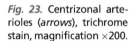
Fig. 23. Centrizonal arterioles (*arrows*), trichrome stain, magnification ×200.

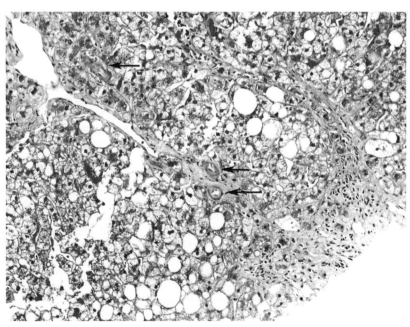

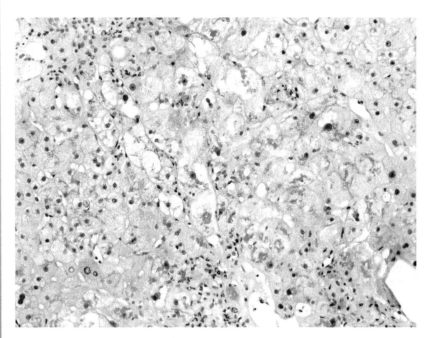

Fig. 24. Amiodarone toxicity with steatohepatitis features, H&E stain, magnification ×200.

by accumulation of drug in lysosomes.[18,19] This leads to hepatocellular and Kupffer cell foamy change. The foamy areas show lamellar lysosomal inclusion bodies on ultrastructural evaluation.[18] Phospholipidosis is not always seen in amiodarone toxicity[18] and is independent of steatohepatitis.[16]

Irinotecan

Irinotecan, a chemotherapeutic agent used preoperatively in patients with colorectal cancer with hepatic metastases, can cause steatohepatitis-like injury to the liver. This has been referred to as chemotherapy-associated steatohepatitis in the oncology literature.[20]

Methotrexate

Methotrexate is a folate antagonist used for long-term treatment of rheumatoid arthritis, psoriasis, and inflammatory bowel disease. Liver toxicity typically manifests as steatosis, anisonucleosis, portal inflammation, and portal-based fibrosis. It may also exacerbate or precipitate steatohepatitis in patients with risk factors such as obesity and diabetes. The risk of liver toxicity is also exacerbated with heavy alcohol use, preexisting liver disease, daily dosing, and a high cumulative dose.[21] Some patients with a high cumulative dose can develop steatohepatitis without metabolic risk factors (**Fig. 25**).[22,23]

Perhexiline Maleate/ Diethylaminoethoxyhexestrol

Perhexiline maleate (Pexid), an antiangina drug, and diethylaminoethoxyhexestrol (Coralgil), a vasodilator, have been used extensively in Europe and Japan, respectively. Both drugs can cause NASH and phospholipidoses similar to amiodarone.[24,25]

Other drugs have been described in association with NAFLD, but the evidence linking them to NASH is less strong. It is unlikely that these drugs have a direct role in causing NASH, but they may precipitate steatohepatitis in the presence of other risk factors.

Other Drugs

Tamoxifen is an antiestrogen drug used in patients with breast cancer. Steatohepatitis risk may only be increased in overweight or obese women.[26] Steroids, estrogen, and diethylstilbestrol often lead to hepatic steatosis, but steatohepatitis is rare.[17,27] Nifedipine is a calcium channel blocker that has been implicated in NASH, but risk factors for NASH are often also present in patients treated with this medication, creating some uncertainty about a definite association between this drug and steatohepatitis.[28]

HEREDITARY HEMOCHROMATOSIS

A mild to moderate hepatocyte siderosis (generally nonzonal) and/or Kupffer cell siderosis has been

Fig. 25. Methotrexate-induced changes with steatosis and portal inflammation (*A*), as well as periportal fibrosis (*B*). H&E and trichrome stains, magnification ×100 to ×200.

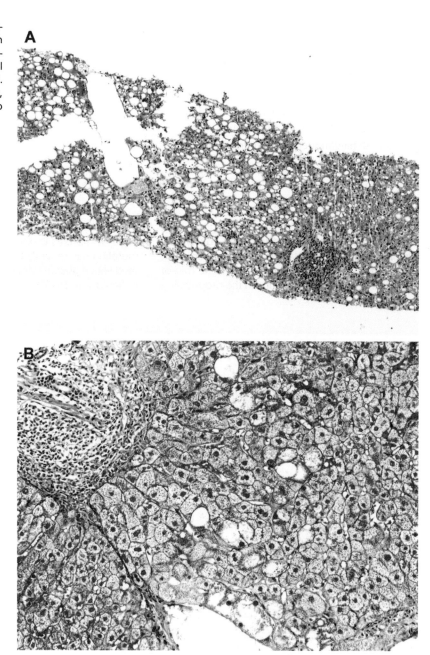

described in up to 21% of patients with NAFLD with known wild-type *HFE*[29] (although only 6% of these patients had isolated hepatocellular iron[29]). Serum ferritin, an acute phase reactant, can be increased in patients with NAFLD, which may result in clinical suspicion for hereditary hemochromatosis. A high serum ferritin level and increased iron saturation, however, may more strongly suggest coexistent hereditary hemochromatosis and, with C282Y *HFE* mutation, which is associated with greater iron deposition in liver tissue, biopsy may be warranted, even in a patient with well-established NASH, to rule out iron overload and associated fibrosis.[1] On iron stain, hereditary hemochromatosis is usually characterized by a more intense iron deposition, predominantly in hepatocytes, which is more pronounced in the periportal region (**Table 7**),

Table 7 Patterns of siderosis in NASH	
Distribution of Iron	**Interpretation**
Pattern 1: KC	Secondary siderosis
Pattern 2: KC and mild/moderate HC (random)	Secondary siderosis
Pattern 3: mild/moderate HC (random)	Secondary siderosis
Pattern 4: mild/moderate HC (periportal)	HH or secondary siderosis
Pattern 5: marked HC (any)	HH or secondary siderosis

Abbreviations: HC, hepatocellular; HH, hereditary hemochromatosis (untreated); KC, Kupffer cell.

although there is some overlap (**Fig. 26**); typical histologic features of NASH are not observed in isolated hereditary hemochromatosis. The role of hepatic iron and *HFE* mutations in the progression of NASH fibrosis is uncertain.[30–32] The H63D *HFE* mutation has recently been reported to be associated with higher steatosis grade and higher NAS in patients with NASH.[29]

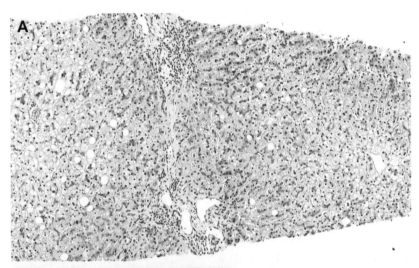

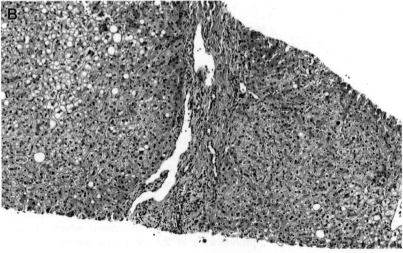

Fig. 26. Siderosis in hereditary hemochromatosis is generally periportal (*A*). Biopsies can have unrelated steatosis (*B*). (*Continued on next page*).

Fig. 26. (continued) Iron deposition in steatohepatitis can look similar to hereditary hemochromatosis (*C*). Secondary siderosis with iron deposition mainly in Kupffer cells (*D*) is not associated with hereditary hemochromatosis and may also be encountered in the setting of NAFLD, usually in a patient with a history of transfusion. H&E and iron stains, magnification ×100 to ×200.

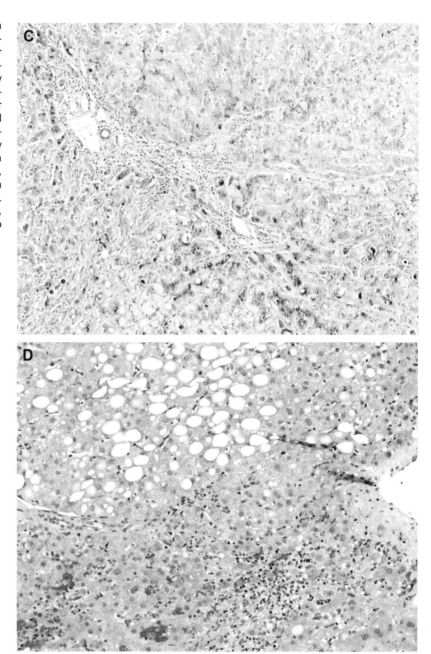

METABOLIC DISORDERS

Several metabolic disorders can show overlapping features with NASH.

Glycogenic Hepatopathy

Glycogenic hepatopathy develops in diabetic patients with poor glycemic control and is characterized by swollen hepatocytes and glycogenated nuclei similar to NASH. However, it occurs more commonly in type 1 diabetes, as opposed to type 2 diabetes, which is more common in NASH. Numerous megamitochondria can be present in glycogenic hepatopathy; fat, Mallory hyaline, significant inflammation, and pericellular fibrosis are usually absent or inconspicuous (**Fig. 27**).[33]

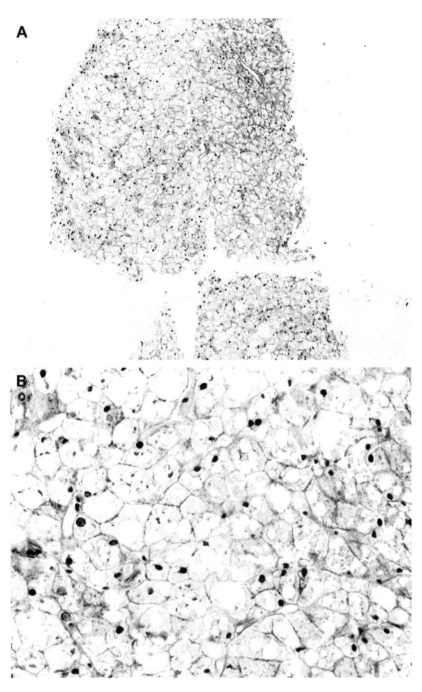

Fig. 27. Glycogenic hepatopathy (*A*) is a pitfall that may be misdiagnosed as steatohepatitis given the swollen cleared out cells, although note the relative lack of steatosis (*A*) and more prominent megamitochondria (*B*). H&E stains, magnification ×100 and ×400.

Diabetic Hepatosclerosis

Diabetic hepatosclerosis is a term used to describe dense nonzonal perisinusoidal fibrosis and basement membrane deposition that occur in patients with long-standing insulin-dependent diabetes (Fig. 28). It is associated with severe microvascular disease in other organs and may represent a form of hepatic microangiopathy.[34] In addition to sinusoidal fibrosis, perivenular fibrosis and hyaline thickening of small hepatic artery branches may be present. Features typical of NASH such as steatosis or hepatocellular ballooning are not seen.

Fig. 28. Diabetic hepato-sclerosis is a pitfall that may be misdiagnosed as steatohepatitis given similar pericellular hyaline material that may be mistaken for pericellular fibrosis of steatohepatitis. Magnification ×400.

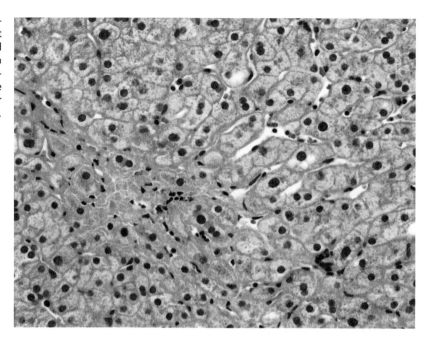

These patients often have an increased level of alkaline phosphatase, an unusual finding for NASH.

Wilson Disease

Wilson disease is often associated with steatosis and glycogenated nuclei (**Fig. 29**). In some cases, swollen hepatocytes and Mallory hyaline can be present and can mimic steatohepatitis. The nonzonal distribution of fat and Mallory hyaline in Wilson disease, a chronic hepatitis-like pattern of inflammation, and portal-based fibrosis are helpful in the differential diagnosis because these findings are unusual in NASH. In addition, it is unusual for Wilson disease to present after age 55 (years), so this consideration can be excluded in an older patient. In difficult cases, quantitative copper determination from urine and/or paraffin-embedded liver tissue can allow for definitive diagnosis. Note that ceruloplasmin levels may be falsely increased into the normal range in patients with active disease, resulting in a false-negative value. Histochemical copper stains are not reliable in ruling out Wilson disease on biopsy.

MICROVESICULAR STEATOSIS

Pure microvesicular steatosis is a rare phenomenon and does not occur in NASH (**Fig. 30**). It signifies severe mitochondrial injury and is seen in alcoholic foamy liver degeneration, Reyes syndrome (in children), acute fatty liver of pregnancy,

rare genetic diseases (eg, carnitine deficiency), and as an adverse effect of drugs/toxins such as cocaine, tetracycline, valproic acid, and zidovudine. A substantial number of cases of NAFLD have a component of microvesicular steatosis,[35] which has been associated with higher grades of steatosis, ballooning cell injury, presence of Mallory hyaline, megamitochondria, higher NAS, and more advanced fibrosis, although a definite role for microvesicular steatosis in the pathophysiology of NASH-related liver injury remains uncertain.

MORE THAN MILD PORTAL INFLAMMATION

Portal inflammation in steatohepatitis is typically mild (see **Fig. 5**). If prominent portal inflammation is present, other causes such as hepatitis B or C, autoimmune hepatitis, primary biliary cirrhosis, or Wilson disease have to be clinically excluded. The presence of lymphoid aggregates (as in hepatitis C), viral inclusions (as in hepatitis B), numerous plasma cells (as in autoimmune hepatitis), or bile duct injury (as in primary biliary cirrhosis) is unusual in NASH. After other causes have been clinically excluded, the case can be regarded as steatohepatitis with unusually prominent portal inflammation (**Fig. 31**). These cases are likely to be associated with a higher degree of fibrosis.[36]

The presence of autoantibodies does not necessarily signify autoimmune hepatitis, as various serum autoantibodies have been detected in up

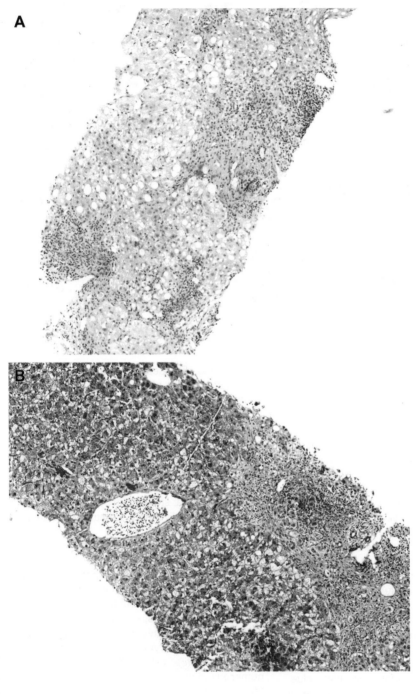

Fig. 29. Wilson disease may be misdiagnosed as steatohepatitis given the presence of fat, inflammation and swollen cells (*A*), but note the more prominent portal inflammation (*A*) and periportal fibrosis (*B*) in 1 case of Wilson disease. (*Continued on next page*).

to 36% of steatohepatitis patients.[37] Antinuclear antibodies and antismooth muscle antibodies have been reported in 20% and 3% to 6% of patients, respectively.[37–39] Both autoantibodies may be present together in rare cases.[37–39] NASH patients with autoantibodies generally show typical histologic features of NASH[39] and probably do not benefit from steroid therapy.[37] Antimitochondrial antibodies have rarely been detected in patients with NASH (∼1%) and are not associated

Fig. 29. (*continued*) Another case of Wilson disease shows swollen cells suspicious for ballooned hepatocytes (*C*) as well as pericellular fibrosis (*D*), although the cholestasis in this biopsy would be unexpected in isolated nonalcoholic steatohepatitis. H&E and trichrome stains, magnification ×100 to ×200.

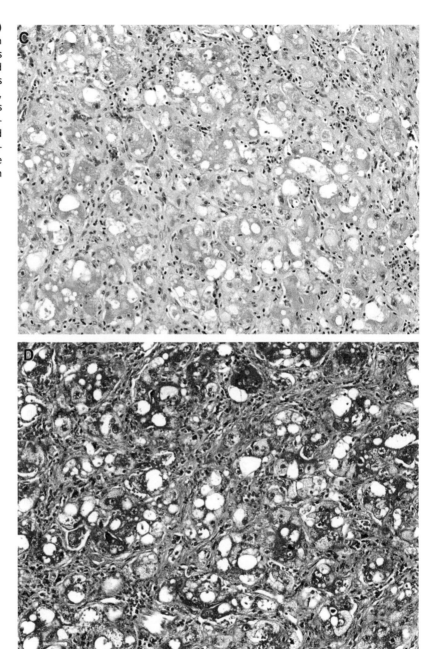

with primary biliary cirrhosis.[37] In all of these studies, the autoantibody titers were generally low, so high titer autoantibodies should raise more concern for another or coexistent etiology. On biopsy, the presence of steatosis, ballooning, and pericellular fibrosis as well as the absence of high liver transaminases, prominent portal inflammation, numerous plasma cells, and prominent hepatocellular damage reliably distinguish steatohepatitis from autoimmune hepatitis.

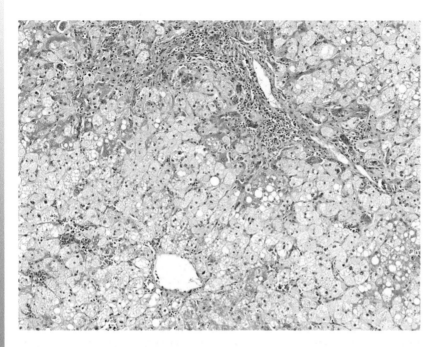

Fig. *30.* Microvesicular steatosis predominates in this case of mitochondrial toxicity, which should not be mistaken for steatohepatitis. H&E stain, magnification ×100.

PEDIATRIC NASH

NASH-related cirrhosis has been described in children as young as 8 years of age (with NAFLD documented as early as 2 years of age).[1,8,40] In 1 study of obese school children, 23% of children aged 17 to 18 years had unexplained increased levels of alanine aminotransferase (>40 IU/L).[40] In addition to obesity, older age, male gender, and Hispanic ethnicity are independent predictors of NAFLD prevalence in children.[1] Currently, aspartate aminotransferase/alanine aminotransferase screening is recommended (in 1 study) for obese children, starting at age 10 (years), with body mass index values in the 85th to 94th percentile and with other risk factors.[41] However, the more recent practice guidelines did not make a formal recommendation for pediatric screening,[1] given

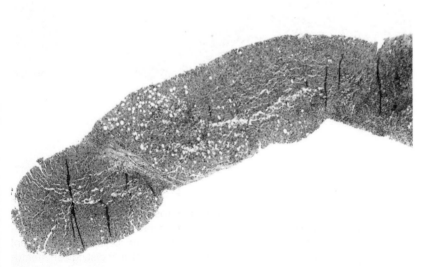

Fig. 31. More than mild portal inflammation in a patient with hepatitis C and mild steatosis, although if viral and other causes are excluded, this degree of portal inflammation does not necessarily exclude consideration of steatohepatitis. H&E stain, magnification ×40.

the lack of sufficient evidence at this time. Current recommendations suggest a need for liver biopsy in children when NAFLD is suspected but the diagnosis is unclear, or before starting hepatotoxic medicines or pharmacologic therapy for NASH.[1]

The histologic features of NASH in children may differ from adult NASH. It has been proposed that pediatric steatohepatitis can be classified into 2 types based on histologic features.

Type 1 NASH

Type 1 NASH resembles adult NASH with zone 3 predominance of steatosis, hepatocellular ballooning, and fibrosis.[8]

Type 2 NASH

In type 2 NASH, steatosis is often severe and may lack zone 3 predominance (Fig. 32). Ballooned hepatocytes, Mallory hyaline, and acinar inflammation may be mild or absent, whereas portal-based chronic inflammation may be prominent. Portal-based fibrosis in the absence of pericentral/sinusoidal fibrosis can occur (ie, stage 1C, see Table 5).[8] Some adults may also show this pattern of NASH injury, but the finding is rare (only 3 out of 288 adult biopsies evaluated by the NASH CRN) and not related to gender or race/ethnicity differences.[42] The differential diagnosis may include other hepatitic causes, such as autoimmune hepatitis, but severe steatosis should raise suspicion for type 2 NASH in this scenario and result in clinical correlation.

Most pediatric patients with NASH in 1 series showed type 2 features,[8] whereas mixed type 1 and type 2 features were seen in most cases in another study.[43] The pathology report in cases with type 2 features should reflect that the classic criteria for steatohepatitis are not fulfilled (as occurs in many pediatric cases), but that it may be prudent to manage the patient as appropriate for steatohepatitis.

Genetic and Metabolic Liver Disease

Children younger than age 2 (years) with fatty liver should be evaluated for rare genetic disorders such as fatty acid oxidation defects, lysosomal storage disorders, and peroxisomal disorders.[1] Fatty acid oxidation defects typically manifest with microvesicular steatosis and possibly also with ductular reaction, cholestasis, and fibrosis.[44] Abetalipoproteinemia and familial hypobetalipoproteinemia may also present with steatosis in young patients and some patients with abetalipoproteinemia have reportedly developed progressive fibrosis.[45] Other disorders of lipoprotein and lipid metabolism (eg, familial high-density lipoprotein deficiency (Tangier disease), familial hypercholesterolemia, Wolman disease, ceramidase deficiency (Farber disease), glycosyl ceramide lipidosis (Gaucher disease), and sphingomyelin-cholesterol lipidosis (Niemann-Pick

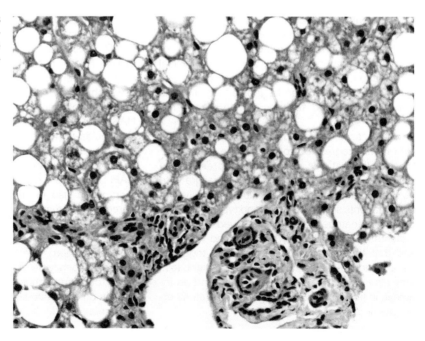

Fig. 32. Severe steatosis in a periportal to panacinar distribution in a case of NASH. H&E stain, magnification ×400.

disease)) may variably demonstrate vacuolated/foamy change in the liver, predominantly in Kupffer cells (consisting of products related to lipoprotein and lipid metabolism).[46–53] Although lipogranulomas are common in NASH, diffuse Kupffer cell foamy change is not a feature of NAFLD and suggests a storage disorder. Hereditary tyrosinemia is a genetic disease with features of steatohepatitis and demonstrates steatosis with pericellular fibrosis but also prominent hepatocanalicular cholestasis and possibly also hepatocellular dysplasia.[54] Cystic fibrosis changes may also include hepatic steatosis and periportal fibrosis, but with ductular reaction and dilatation (possibly with inspissated secretions), and possibly with progression to multilobular biliary cirrhosis.[55]

Familial NASH refers to identification of NASH (or cryptogenic cirrhosis) in high frequency within several kindreds in whom obesity and type 2 diabetes mellitus are prevalent,[56] which suggests a common mechanism of disease and perhaps also some heritable risk. A steatohepatitis pattern of injury has also been described in

- Partial lipodystrophy[57]
- Bardet-Biedl syndrome[58]
- Alstrom syndrome[59]
- Bloom syndrome[60]

Prominent steatosis, without fibrosis, has also been noted in Dorfman-Chanarin syndrome.[61,62]

STEATOHEPATITIS WITH AN ACUTE/SUBACUTE PRESENTATION

Most patients with NASH are diagnosed as a result of an asymptomatic increase in liver transaminase levels, the presence of steatosis on imaging, or incidental hepatomegaly on a routine physical examination. Some patients can also present with cirrhosis, which can be labeled cryptogenic if typical histologic features of NASH are not present.

In rare cases, a subacute to acute presentation with rapid progression to liver failure can occur. Most of the patients with an acute presentation are obese women with onset of liver failure 4 to 16 weeks after initial presentation.[63] The liver in these patients shows cirrhosis and typical features of active steatohepatitis. It is believed that these patients develop silent cirrhosis related to NASH and that the subacute presentation is triggered by an additional liver injury. Rapid weight loss may also possibly precipitate NASH[64] and an increase in fibrosis has been reported in 1 study after gastric bypass surgery.[65]

PROGNOSIS AND TREATMENT

NAFLD is associated with increased mortality, most commonly as a result of cardiovascular disease, and NASH has an increased liver-related mortality rate.[1,9,66–73] Patients with NASH cirrhosis may develop HCC, but at a lower rate than patients with hepatitis C,[74,75] and overall, NASH cirrhosis reportedly has a lower rate of decompensation and mortality versus patients with hepatitis C cirrhosis.[74] Nevertheless, overall mortality is similar to hepatitis C (ie, 10-year survival is 81.5%).[75]

Management of NAFLD requires attention to risk factors with emphasis on weight loss, diet, exercise, and improved control of diabetes.[1] Weight loss usually reduces hepatic steatosis after a 3% to 5% reduction in weight.[76] More significant weight loss (>10%) seems necessary to reduce histologic evidence of liver injury.[76,77] Exercise alone, without weight loss, may improve steatosis, but any effects on liver injury are unknown.[78,79] Some murine research has implicated a possible role for particular dietary constituents in NASH, such as trans fats.[80]

Clinical trials are ongoing and treatment choices are evolving. For example, metformin (a biguanide, which may act as an insulin-sensitizing agent) is no longer recommended as a specific NASH treatment[1,81]; vitamin E (an antioxidant) is considered a first-line pharmacotherapy for nondiabetic adults with biopsy proven NASH.[82] Children with NAFLD may have a diet low in vitamin E, which may contribute to NAFLD pathophysiology in this population,[83] although vitamin E therapy has not proved to be efficacious in this group.[84] Pioglitazone (a thiazolidinedione, which may act through PPAR-γ receptors) may be used to treat biopsy proven NASH, but long-term safety and efficacy have not been established.[1,2,82] Ursodeoxycholic acid (a bile acid with a variety of potential actions) is also not recommended for treatment of NASH.[1,85] The benefit of treatment with omega-3 fatty acids (polyunsaturated fatty acids) remains unknown, though omega-3 fatty acids may be used to treat hypertriglyceridemia in patients with NAFLD and there is some preliminary support for therapeutic use in NAFLD.[1,86] Bariatric surgery (foregut type) may be considered in patients with NAFLD without cirrhosis,[1] but safety and efficacy in the setting of cirrhosis (due to NAFLD) is not well established.[1,87,88] Statins (3-hydroxy-3-methylglutaryl-coenzyme A reductase inhibitors that lower total serum cholesterol and low-density lipoprotein concentrations) may be used to treat dyslipidemia in patients with NAFLD, but should not

Fig. 33. Hepatocellular adenoma arising in background fatty liver, H&E stain (*A*) and positive labeling on a serum amyloid A immunohistochemical stain, consistent with an inflammatory variant (*B*), magnification ×100.

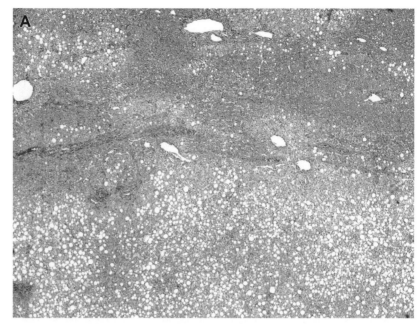

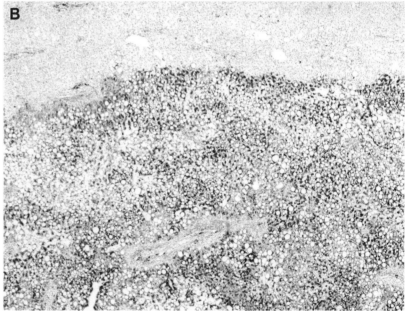

be used to specifically treat NASH at this time.[1] Patients with NASH cirrhosis should be screened for esophageal varices and possibly for HCC.[1,89,90] Patients transplanted for NASH with HCC have had less aggressive tumor features (eg, less frequent vascular invasion and poorly differentiated foci), and long recurrence-free survival compared with patients with HCC in hepatitis C cirrhosis.[91] Recent data have also indicated that hepatocellular adenomas, especially the inflammatory variant, occur commonly in obese and diabetic patients (**Fig. 33**).[92,93]

ACKNOWLEDGMENTS

The authors thank Dr. Linda Ferrell for her comments on the manuscript.

REFERENCES

1. Chalasani N, Younossi Z, Lavine JE, et al. The diagnosis and management of non-alcoholic fatty liver disease: practice guideline by the American Association for the Study of Liver Diseases, American College of Gastroenterology, and the American Gastroenterological Association. Am J Gastroenterol 2012;107(6):811–26.

2. Vernon G, Baranova A, Younossi ZM. Systematic review: the epidemiology and natural history of non-alcoholic fatty liver disease and non-alcoholic steatohepatitis in adults. Aliment Pharmacol Ther 2011;34(3):274–85.

3. Saadeh S, Younossi ZM, Remer EM, et al. The utility of radiological imaging in nonalcoholic fatty liver disease. Gastroenterology 2002;123(3):745–50.

4. Neuschwander-Tetri BA, Caldwell SH. Nonalcoholic steatohepatitis: summary of an AASLD Single Topic Conference. Hepatology 2003;37(5):1202–19.

5. Kleiner DE, Brunt EM, Van Natta M, et al. Design and validation of a histological scoring system for nonalcoholic fatty liver disease. Hepatology 2005;41(6):1313–21.

6. Batts KP, Ludwig J. Chronic hepatitis. An update on terminology and reporting. Am J Surg Pathol 1995;19(12):1409–17.

7. Brunt EM, Janney CG, Di Bisceglie AM, et al. Nonalcoholic steatohepatitis: a proposal for grading and staging the histological lesions. Am J Gastroenterol 1999;94(9):2467–74.

8. Schwimmer JB, Behling C, Newbury R, et al. Histopathology of pediatric nonalcoholic fatty liver disease. Hepatology 2005;42(3):641–9.

9. Matteoni CA, Younossi ZM, Gramlich T, et al. Nonalcoholic fatty liver disease: a spectrum of clinical and pathological severity. Gastroenterology 1999;116(6):1413–9.

10. Guy CD, Suzuki A, Burchette JL, et al. Costaining for keratins 8/18 plus ubiquitin improves detection of hepatocyte injury in nonalcoholic fatty liver disease. Hum Pathol 2012;43(6):790–800.

11. Lackner C, Gogg-Kamerer M, Zatloukal K, et al. Ballooned hepatocytes in steatohepatitis: the value of keratin immunohistochemistry for diagnosis. J Hepatol 2008;48(5):821–8.

12. Caldwell SH, Oelsner DH, Iezzoni JC, et al. Cryptogenic cirrhosis: clinical characterization and risk factors for underlying disease. Hepatology 1999;29(3):664–9.

13. Gill RM, Belt P, Wilson L, et al. Centrizonal arteries and microvessels in nonalcoholic steatohepatitis. Am J Surg Pathol 2011;35(9):1400–4.

14. Stravitz RT, Sanyal AJ. Drug-induced steatohepatitis. Clin Liver Dis 2003;7(2):435–51.

15. Raja K, Thung SN, Fiel MI, et al. Drug-induced steatohepatitis leading to cirrhosis: long-term toxicity of amiodarone use. Semin Liver Dis 2009;29(4):423–8.

16. Guigui B, Perrot S, Berry JP, et al. Amiodarone-induced hepatic phospholipidosis: a morphological alteration independent of pseudoalcoholic liver disease. Hepatology 1988;8(5):1063–8.

17. Ramachandran R, Kakar S. Histological patterns in drug-induced liver disease. J Clin Pathol 2009;62(6):481–92.

18. Lewis JH, Mullick F, Ishak KG, et al. Histopathologic analysis of suspected amiodarone hepatotoxicity. Hum Pathol 1990;21(1):59–67.

19. Richer M, Robert S. Fatal hepatotoxicity following oral administration of amiodarone. Ann Pharmacother 1995;29(6):582–6.

20. Pawlik TM, Olino K, Gleisner AL, et al. Preoperative chemotherapy for colorectal liver metastases: impact on hepatic histology and postoperative outcome. J Gastrointest Surg 2007;11(7):860–8.

21. Langman G, Hall PM, Todd G. Role of non-alcoholic steatohepatitis in methotrexate-induced liver injury. J Gastroenterol Hepatol 2001;16(12):1395–401.

22. Berends MA, van Oijen MG, Snoek J, et al. Reliability of the Roenigk classification of liver damage after methotrexate treatment for psoriasis: a clinicopathologic study of 160 liver biopsy specimens. Arch Dermatol 2007;143(12):1515–9.

23. Roenigk HH Jr, Auerbach R, Maibach HI, et al. Methotrexate guidelines–revised. J Am Acad Dermatol 1982;6(2):145–55.

24. Kubo M, Hostetler KY. Metabolic basis of diethylaminoethoxyhexestrol-induced phospholipid fatty liver. Am J Physiol 1987;252(3 Pt 1):E375–9.

25. Lewis D, Wainwright HC, Kew MC, et al. Liver damage associated with perhexiline maleate. Gut 1979;20(3):186–9.

26. Bruno S, Maisonneuve P, Castellana P, et al. Incidence and risk factors for non-alcoholic steatohepatitis: prospective study of 5408 women enrolled in Italian tamoxifen chemoprevention trial. BMJ 2005;330(7497):932.

27. Steinberg H, Webb WM, Rafsky HA. Hepatomegaly with fatty infiltration secondary to cortisone therapy: case report. Gastroenterology 1952;21(2):304–9.

28. Babany G, Uzzan F, Larrey D, et al. Alcoholic-like liver lesions induced by nifedipine. J Hepatol 1989;9(2):252–5.

29. Nelson JE, Brunt EM, Kowdley KV. Lower serum hepcidin and greater parenchymal iron in nonalcoholic fatty liver disease patients with C282Y HFE mutations. Hepatology 2012;56(5):1730–40.

30. George DK, Powell LW, Losowsky MS. The haemochromatosis gene: a co-factor for chronic liver

diseases? J Gastroenterol Hepatol 1999;14(8): 745–9.

31. Chitturi S, Weltman M, Farrell GC, et al. HFE mutations, hepatic iron, and fibrosis: ethnic-specific association of NASH with C282Y but not with fibrotic severity. Hepatology 2002;36(1):142–9.

32. Fargion S, Mattioli M, Fracanzani AL, et al. Hyperferritinemia, iron overload, and multiple metabolic alterations identify patients at risk for nonalcoholic steatohepatitis. Am J Gastroenterol 2001;96(8): 2448–55.

33. Torbenson M, Chen YY, Brunt E, et al. Glycogenic hepatopathy: an underrecognized hepatic complication of diabetes mellitus. Am J Surg Pathol 2006;30(4):508–13.

34. Harrison SA, Brunt EM, Goodman ZD, et al. Diabetic hepatosclerosis: diabetic microangiopathy of the liver. Arch Pathol Lab Med 2006;130(1): 27–32.

35. Tandra S, Yeh MM, Brunt EM, et al. Presence and significance of microvesicular steatosis in nonalcoholic fatty liver disease. J Hepatol 2011;55(3): 654–9.

36. Brunt EM. Histopathology of non-alcoholic fatty liver disease. Clin Liver Dis 2009;13(4):533–44.

37. Loria P, Lonardo A, Leonardi F, et al. Non-organ-specific autoantibodies in nonalcoholic fatty liver disease: prevalence and correlates. Dig Dis Sci 2003;48(11):2173–81.

38. Adams LA, Lindor KD, Angulo P. The prevalence of autoantibodies and autoimmune hepatitis in patients with nonalcoholic fatty liver disease. Am J Gastroenterol 2004;99(7):1316–20.

39. Cotler SJ, Kanji K, Keshavarzian A, et al. Prevalence and significance of autoantibodies in patients with non-alcoholic steatohepatitis. J Clin Gastroenterol 2004;38(9):801–4.

40. Schwimmer JB, Deutsch R, Kahen T, et al. Prevalence of fatty liver in children and adolescents. Pediatrics 2006;118(4):1388–93.

41. Barlow SE. Expert committee recommendations regarding the prevention, assessment, and treatment of child and adolescent overweight and obesity: summary report. Pediatrics 2007;120(Suppl 4):S164–92.

42. Kleiner DE, Behling C, Brunt E, et al. Comparison of adult and pediatric NAFLD - confirmation of a second pattern of progressive fatty liver disease in children. Hepatology 2006;44(Suppl):259A.

43. Nobili V, Marcellini M, Devito R, et al. NAFLD in children: a prospective clinical-pathological study and effect of lifestyle advice. Hepatology 2006;44(2): 458–65.

44. Bioulac-Sage P, Parrot-Roulaud F, Mazat JP, et al. Fatal neonatal liver failure and mitochondrial cytopathy (oxidative phosphorylation deficiency): a light and electron microscopic study of the liver. Hepatology 1993;18(4):839–46.

45. Partin JS, Partin JC, Schubert WK, et al. Liver ultrastructure in abetalipoproteinemia: evolution of micronodular cirrhosis. Gastroenterology 1974;67(1): 107–18.

46. Bale PM, Clifton-Bligh P, Benjamin BN, et al. Pathology of Tangier disease. J Clin Pathol 1971;24(7): 609–16.

47. Dechelotte P, Kantelip B, de Laguillaumie BV, et al. Tangier disease. A histological and ultrastructural study. Pathol Res Pract 1985;180(4):424–30.

48. Pagani F, Pariyarath R, Garcia R, et al. New lysosomal acid lipase gene mutants explain the phenotype of Wolman disease and cholesteryl ester storage disease. J Lipid Res 1998;39(7):1382–8.

49. Antonarakis SE, Valle D, Moser HW, et al. Phenotypic variability in siblings with Farber disease. J Pediatr 1984;104(3):406–9.

50. Lachmann RH, Wight DG, Lomas DJ, et al. Massive hepatic fibrosis in Gaucher's disease: clinicopathological and radiological features. QJM 2000; 93(4):237–44.

51. Niemann A. Ein unbekanntes Krankenheitsbild. Jahrbuch für Kinderheilkunde 1914;79:1–10 [in German].

52. Pick L. Uber die lipoidzellige splenhepatomegalie typus Niemann-Pick als Stoffwechselerkrankung. Med Klin 1927;23:1483–8 [in German].

53. Buja LM, Kovanen PT, Bilheimer DW. Cellular pathology of homozygous familial hypercholesterolemia. Am J Pathol 1979;97(2):327–57.

54. Dehner LP, Snover DC, Sharp HL, et al. Hereditary tyrosinemia type I (chronic form): pathologic findings in the liver. Hum Pathol 1989;20(2): 149–58.

55. Craig JM, Haddad H, Shwachman H. The pathological changes in the liver in cystic fibrosis of the pancreas. AMA J Dis Child 1957;93(4):357–69.

56. Struben VM, Hespenheide EE, Caldwell SH. Nonalcoholic steatohepatitis and cryptogenic cirrhosis within kindreds. Am J Med 2000;108(1):9–13.

57. Powell EE, Searle J, Mortimer R. Steatohepatitis associated with limb lipodystrophy. Gastroenterology 1989;97(4):1022–4.

58. Sahu JK, Jain V. Laurence-Moon-Bardet-Biedl syndrome. JNMA J Nepal Med Assoc 2008;47(172): 235–7.

59. Awazu M, Tanaka T, Sato S, et al. Hepatic dysfunction in two sibs with Alstrom syndrome: case report and review of the literature. Am J Med Genet 1997; 69(1):13–6.

60. Wang J, Cornford ME, German J, et al. Sclerosing hyaline necrosis of the liver in Bloom syndrome. Arch Pathol Lab Med 1999;123(4):346–50.

61. Gurakan F, Kaymaz F, Kocak N, et al. A cause of fatty liver: neutral lipid storage disease with ichthyosis–electron microscopic findings. Dig Dis Sci 1999;44(11):2214–7.

62. Mela D, Artom A, Goretti R, et al. Dorfman-Chanarin syndrome: a case with prevalent hepatic involvement. J Hepatol 1996;25(5):769–71.

63. Caldwell SH, Hespenheide EE. Subacute liver failure in obese women. Am J Gastroenterol 2002; 97(8):2058–62.

64. Powell EE, Cooksley WG, Hanson R, et al. The natural history of nonalcoholic steatohepatitis: a follow-up study of forty-two patients for up to 21 years. Hepatology 1990;11(1):74–80.

65. Mathurin P, Hollebecque A, Arnalsteen L, et al. Prospective study of the long-term effects of bariatric surgery on liver injury in patients without advanced disease. Gastroenterology 2009;137(2):532–40.

66. Adams LA, Lymp JF, St Sauver J, et al. The natural history of nonalcoholic fatty liver disease: a population-based cohort study. Gastroenterology 2005;129(1):113–21.

67. Dam-Larsen S, Franzmann M, Andersen IB, et al. Long term prognosis of fatty liver: risk of chronic liver disease and death. Gut 2004;53(5):750–5.

68. Ekstedt M, Franzen LE, Mathiesen UL, et al. Long-term follow-up of patients with NAFLD and elevated liver enzymes. Hepatology 2006;44(4):865–73.

69. Dunn W, Xu R, Wingard DL, et al. Suspected nonalcoholic fatty liver disease and mortality risk in a population-based cohort study. Am J Gastroenterol 2008;103(9):2263–71.

70. Rafiq N, Bai C, Fang Y, et al. Long-term follow-up of patients with nonalcoholic fatty liver. Clin Gastroenterol Hepatol 2009;7(2):234–8.

71. Dam-Larsen S, Becker U, Franzmann MB, et al. Final results of a long-term, clinical follow-up in fatty liver patients. Scand J Gastroenterol 2009;44(10): 1236–43.

72. Stepanova M, Rafiq N, Younossi ZM. Components of metabolic syndrome are independent predictors of mortality in patients with chronic liver disease: a population-based study. Gut 2010;59(10):1410–5.

73. Soderberg C, Stal P, Askling J, et al. Decreased survival of subjects with elevated liver function tests during a 28-year follow-up. Hepatology 2010;51(2):595–602.

74. Sanyal AJ, Banas C, Sargeant C, et al. Similarities and differences in outcomes of cirrhosis due to nonalcoholic steatohepatitis and hepatitis C. Hepatology 2006;43(4):682–9.

75. Yatsuji S, Hashimoto E, Tobari M, et al. Clinical features and outcomes of cirrhosis due to non-alcoholic steatohepatitis compared with cirrhosis caused by chronic hepatitis C. J Gastroenterol Hepatol 2009;24(2):248–54.

76. Harrison SA, Fecht W, Brunt EM, et al. Orlistat for overweight subjects with nonalcoholic steatohepatitis: a randomized, prospective trial. Hepatology 2009;49(1):80–6.

77. Promrat K, Kleiner DE, Niemeier HM, et al. Randomized controlled trial testing the effects of weight loss on nonalcoholic steatohepatitis. Hepatology 2010;51(1):121–9.

78. Shojaee-Moradie F, Baynes KC, Pentecost C, et al. Exercise training reduces fatty acid availability and improves the insulin sensitivity of glucose metabolism. Diabetologia 2007;50(2):404–13.

79. Johnson LG, Collier KE, Edwards DJ, et al. Improvement in aerobic capacity after an exercise program in sporadic inclusion body myositis. J Clin Neuromuscul Dis 2009;10(4):178–84.

80. Neuschwander-Tetri BA, Ford DA, Acharya S, et al. Dietary trans-fatty acid induced NASH is normalized following loss of trans-fatty acids from hepatic lipid pools. Lipids 2012;47(10):941–50.

81. Haukeland JW, Konopski Z, Eggesbo HB, et al. Metformin in patients with non-alcoholic fatty liver disease: a randomized, controlled trial. Scand J Gastroenterol 2009;44(7):853–60.

82. Sanyal AJ, Chalasani N, Kowdley KV, et al. Pioglitazone, vitamin E, or placebo for non-alcoholic steatohepatitis. N Engl J Med 2010; 362(18):1675–85.

83. Vos MB, Colvin R, Belt P, et al. Correlation of vitamin E, uric acid, and diet composition with histologic features of pediatric NAFLD. J Pediatr Gastroenterol Nutr 2012;54(1):90–6.

84. Lavine JE, Schwimmer JB, Van Natta ML, et al. Effect of vitamin E or metformin for treatment of nonalcoholic fatty liver disease in children and adolescents: the TONIC randomized controlled trial. JAMA 2011;305(16):1659–68.

85. Lindor KD, Kowdley KV, Heathcote EJ, et al. Ursodeoxycholic acid for treatment of nonalcoholic steatohepatitis: results of a randomized trial. Hepatology 2004;39(3):770–8.

86. Masterton GS, Plevris JN, Hayes PC. Review article: omega-3 fatty acids - a promising novel therapy for non-alcoholic fatty liver disease. Aliment Pharmacol Ther 2010;31(7):679–92.

87. Mummadi RR, Kasturi KS, Chennareddygari S, et al. Effect of bariatric surgery on nonalcoholic fatty liver disease: systematic review and meta-analysis. Clin Gastroenterol Hepatol 2008;6(12): 1396–402.

88. Chavez-Tapia NC, Tellez-Avila FI, Barrientos-Gutierrez T, et al. Bariatric surgery for non-alcoholic steatohepatitis in obese patients. Cochrane Database Syst Rev 2010;(1):CD007340.

89. Garcia-Tsao G, Sanyal AJ, Grace ND, et al. Prevention and management of gastroesophageal varices and variceal hemorrhage in cirrhosis. Am J Gastroenterol 2007;102(9):2086–102.

90. Bruix J, Sherman M. Management of hepatocellular carcinoma: an update. Hepatology 2011;53(3): 1020–2.

91. Hernandez-Alejandro R, Croome KP, Drage M, et al. A comparison of survival and pathologic features of non-alcoholic steatohepatitis and hepatitis C virus patients with hepatocellular carcinoma. World J Gastroenterol 2012;18(31): 4145–9.

92. Bioulac-Sage P, Laumonier H, Laurent C, et al. Hepatocellular adenoma: what is new in 2008. Hepatol Int 2008;2(3):316–21.

93. Bioulac-Sage P, Taouji S, Possenti L, et al. Hepatocellular adenoma subtypes: the impact of overweight and obesity. Liver Int 2012;32(8):1217–21.

Autoimmune Hepatitis

Cristina D. Cole, MD, Romil Saxena, MBBS, MD*

KEYWORDS

• Autoimmune hepatitis • Chronic hepatitis • Overlap syndrome • Interface hepatitis • Autoantibodies
• Diagnostic criteria • Histology • Differential diagnosis

ABSTRACT

Autoimmune hepatitis is a chronic necroinflammatory disease of unknown cause that is characterized by increased aminotransferases, autoantibodies, increased immunoglobulin G levels, and histologic interface hepatitis. Diagnostic criteria have been developed to aid in the differentiation from other liver disorders. Liver biopsy is an essential part of the diagnostic criteria and is also crucial to the management of the disease. This article presents an updated review of the diagnosis of autoimmune hepatitis, focusing on the microscopic features of the disease and their differential diagnosis. An overview of the variant phenotypes of autoimmune hepatitis, including overlap syndromes, is also presented.

Pathologic Key Features
OF AUTOIMMUNE HEPATITIS

1. The hallmark of autoimmune hepatitis is interface hepatitis with lymphoplasmacytic infiltrates and varying degrees of lobular inflammation and damage.

2. Additional helpful features include hepatocyte rosette formation, emperipolesis, giant syncytial hepatocytes, and a lack of changes suggesting a different cause.

3. Acute-onset autoimmune hepatitis is characterized by panacinar hepatitis and/or centrilobular perivenulitis with or without interface activity.

4. Approximately 36% of patients with autoimmune hepatitis are cirrhotic at the time of presentation.

OVERVIEW

Autoimmune hepatitis (AIH) is a chronic necroinflammatory disease of unknown cause that is characterized by increased aminotransferases, autoantibodies, increased immunoglobulin G (IgG) levels, and histologic interface hepatitis. AIH has an incidence of 1 to 2/100,000 per year and a prevalence of 10 to 20/100,000.[1] It affects children and adults of all ethnicities and races, but is predominantly a female disorder with peak incidences in adolescence and again at ages 35 to 40 years.[1] A recent population-based survey found that 72% of cases are diagnosed in patients after age 40 years.[2] The presentation of AIH is highly variable and ranges from an asymptomatic increase of aminotransferases, to acute fulminant liver failure, to cirrhosis. Associations with other autoimmune diseases such as autoimmune thyroiditis, inflammatory bowel disease, rheumatoid arthritis, Graves disease, and celiac disease are common.[1] The clinical, laboratory, and histologic manifestations of AIH are found in a diverse group of acute and chronic liver diseases, and consequently the diagnosis of AIH requires the definitive exclusion of other causative factors. The examination of liver tissue is an essential component in this discriminative process.

DIAGNOSIS OF AIH

It is well recognized that timely and appropriate treatment of AIH leads to favorable short-term and long-term outcomes in most patients, although untreated disease confers a poor prognosis.[3] Because undiagnosed AIH means untreated AIH, it is critical for the disease to be identified in a timely

Neither author has any financial interests to disclose.
Department of Pathology and Laboratory Medicine, Indiana University School of Medicine, 350 West 11th Street, Indianapolis, IN 46202, USA
* Corresponding author.
E-mail address: rsaxena@iupui.edu

surgpath.theclinics.com

fashion. However, this can be challenging, in part because AIH does not have a pathognomonic clinical, laboratory, or histologic feature. It is in conditions that lack such a specific and reliable diagnostic test that diagnostic criteria become particularly useful.[4] In 1992, a panel of physicians and pathologists, who became known as the International Autoimmune Hepatitis Group (IAIHG), convened to establish diagnostic criteria for AIH, and in 1998 met again to revise the initial criteria.

Their consensus report included a descriptive set of criteria that could be used in routine clinical practice to diagnose patients as having either definite or probable AIH (Table 1).[5] Definite AIH requires both the exclusion of other conditions that may resemble the disease, as well as the presence of a constellation of histologic and laboratory findings that support its diagnosis. The descriptive criteria are sufficient to diagnose or exclude definite or probable AIH in most patients.[6]

Table 1
Revised diagnostic criteria of the IAIHG

Features	Definite AIH	Probable AIH
Liver histology	Interface hepatitis of moderate or severe activity with or without lobular hepatitis or central-portal bridging necrosis, but without biliary lesions or well-defined granulomas or other prominent changes suggesting a different cause	Same as for definite AIH
Serum biochemistry	Any abnormality in serum aminotransferases, especially if the serum alkaline phosphatase is not markedly increased. Normal serum concentrations of alpha-antitrypsin, copper, and ceruloplasmin	Same as for definite AIH, but patients with abnormal serum concentrations of copper or ceruloplasmin may be included, provided that Wilson disease has been excluded by appropriate investigations
Serum immunoglobulins	Total serum globulin or gamma globulin or IgG concentrations greater than 1.5 times the upper normal limit	Any increase of serum globulin or gamma globulin or IgG concentrations more than the upper normal limit
Serum autoantibodies	Seropositivity for ANA, SMA, or LKM-1 antibodies at titers greater than 1:80. Lower titers (particularly of anti-LKM-1) may be significant in children. Seronegativity for AMA	Same as for definite AIH but at titers of 1:40 or greater. Patients who are seronegative for these antibodies but who are seropositive for other antibodies specified in the text may be included
Viral markers	Seronegativity for markers of current infection with hepatitis A, B, and C viruses	Same as for definite AIH
Other causal factors	Average alcohol consumption less than 25 g/d. No history of recent use of known hepatotoxic drugs	Alcohol consumption less than 50 g/d and no recent use of known hepatotoxic drugs. Patients who have consumed larger amounts of alcohol or who have recently taken potentially hepatotoxic drugs may be included if there is clear evidence of continuing liver damage after abstinence from alcohol or withdrawal of the drug

Abbreviations: AMA, antimitochondrial antibody; ANA, antinuclear antibody; LKM-1, liver kidney microsome-1 antibody; SMA, smooth muscle antibody.

Adapted from Alvarez F, Berg PA, Bianchi FB, et al. International Autoimmune Hepatitis Group Report: review of criteria for diagnosis of autoimmune hepatitis. J Hepatol 1999;31:929–38.

Diagnostic Criteria

The IAIHG report also provided a diagnostic scoring system, created as a research tool to ensure the comparability of study populations in clinical trials, but that could also be applied to diagnostically challenging or atypical cases (Table 2).[5] The scoring system has been shown to have a high sensitivity (97%–100%) for AIH[5]; however, its complexity (13 components) and awkwardness as an easily applicable clinical tool are major drawbacks. To attempt to resolve these limitations, the IAIHG developed simplified diagnostic criteria in 2008 based on only 4 parameters: serum autoantibodies, serum IgG levels, liver histology, and absence of viral hepatitis (Table 3).[7] Demonstration of hepatitis on histology is an integral part of the simplified criteria, reaffirming the importance of liver biopsy in the diagnosis of AIH. Several studies have confirmed the usefulness of these new criteria in various cohorts of

Table 2
Revised scoring system of the IAIHG

Parameter/Feature	Score	Parameter/Feature	Score
Female sex	+2	Drug history:	
ALP:AST (or ALT) ratio:		Positive	−4
<1.5	+2	Negative	+1
1.5–3.0	0	Average alcohol intake:	
>3.0	−2	<25 g/day	+2
Serum globulins *or* IgG level above normal:		>60 g/day	−2
>2.0	+3	Liver histology:	
1.5–2.0	+2	Interface hepatitis	+3
1.0–1.5	+1	Predominantly lymphoplasmacytic	+1
<1.0	0	Rosettes	+1
ANA, SMA, or LKM-1 titers:		None of the above	−5
>1:80	+3	Biliary changes	−3
1:80	+2	Features suggesting a different etiology	−3
1:40	+1	Other autoimmune disease(s)	+2
<1:40	0	HLA DR3 or DR4	+1
AMA positive	−4	Seropositivity for other autoantibodies:	
Hepatitis viral markers:		Includes pANCA, anti-LC1, anti-SLA, anti-actin	+2
Positive	−3	Response to therapy:	
Negative	+3	Complete	+2
		Relapse	+3

Interpretation of Aggregate Scores:
Pre-treatment:
Definite AIH: >15
Probable AIH: 10–15
Post-treatment:
Definite AIH: >17
Probable AIH: 12–17

Abbreviations: ALP, alkaline phosphatase; ALT, alanine aminotransferase; AST, aspartate aminotransferase; HLA, human leukocyte antigen; LC1, liver cytosol type 1 antibody; pANCA, perinuclear antineutrophil cytoplasmic antibody; SLA, soluble liver antigen antibody.

Adapted from Alvarez F, Berg PA, Bianchi FB, et al. International Autoimmune Hepatitis Group Report: review of criteria for diagnosis of autoimmune hepatitis. J Hepatol 1999;31:929–38.

Table 3
Simplified diagnostic criteria of the IAIHG

Parameter/Feature	Cutoff	Score
Autoantibodies[a]:		
ANA or SMA	≥1:40	+1
ANA or SMA	≥1:80	+2
LKM-1	≥1:40	+2
SLA	Positive	+2
IgG	>Upper limit of normal	+1
	>1.10 × upper limit of normal	+2
Histologic features	Compatible with AIH[b]	+1
	Typical AIH[c]	+2
Absence of viral hepatitis	No	0
	Yes	+2
Pretreatment score	Probable AIH	6
	Definite AIH	≥7

[a] Maximum of 2 points total allowed for autoantibodies.
[b] Compatible with AIH: chronic hepatitis with lymphocytic infiltration without all of the features considered typical.
[c] Typical AIH: (1) interface hepatitis, lymphocytic/lymphoplasmacytic infiltrates in portal tracts and extending into the lobule; (2) emperipolesis (active penetration by one cell into and through a larger cell); (3) hepatic rosette formation (all 3 required).
Adapted from Hennes EM, Zeniya M, Czaja AJ, et al. Simplified criteria for the diagnosis of autoimmune hepatitis. Hepatology 2008;48:169–76.

patients, with a sensitivity and specificity of greater than 90% in most instances.[8–11] One important limitation of the simplified criteria is their inferior diagnostic efficacy in patients with AIH with an acute or fulminant presentation; the original scoring system has been shown to perform better in this subset of patients.[12–15] The United States Acute Liver Failure Study Group recently proposed the first diagnostic criteria for AIH presenting as acute liver failure. These criteria primarily emphasize histopathology, characterized by massive hepatic necrosis, plasma cell-enriched inflammatory infiltrates, portal tract lymphoid aggregates, and central perivenulitis.[16] Their clinical usefulness remains to be determined, but, if validated, the criteria may be useful in identifying a subgroup of patients with acute liver failure who would benefit from timely corticosteroid therapy.

Antibodies in Diagnosis

Autoantibodies are an important component in each of the diagnostic scoring systems mentioned earlier, and are currently the basis for classifying AIH into[5]:

- Type 1 (positive for antinuclear antibody [ANA] and/or smooth muscle antibody [SMA])
- Type 2 (liver kidney microsome-1 [LKM-1] antibody–positive) disease

ANA and SMA rarely coexist with anti–LKM-1, and it is this exclusivity that defines the two distinct subpopulations.[17] Although these three serologic markers have been invaluable in directing the diagnosis of AIH, there has been little evidence to indicate their role in the pathogenesis of the disease,[18] and serum titers have not correlated with disease activity or treatment outcomes.[19] Furthermore, these antibodies are commonly found in other hepatic diseases, including:

- Viral hepatitis
- Alcoholic fatty liver disease
- Nonalcoholic fatty liver disease
- Wilson disease
- Primary biliary cirrhosis
- Primary sclerosing cholangitis

A recent study evaluated the performance of these conventional serologic markers by comparing the results of 265 adults who satisfied diagnostic criteria for AIH with 342 adults with other chronic liver diseases.[20]

- The sensitivities of the serum antibodies for the diagnosis of AIH were poor (ANA, 32%; SMA, 16%; and anti–LKM-1, 1%), and diagnostic accuracy ranged from 56% to 61%.
- The presence of both ANA and SMA had superior sensitivity (43%), specificity (99%), positive predictive value (97%), negative predictive value (69%), and diagnostic accuracy (74%) to either marker alone, and therefore this serologic combination may be the most useful first-line battery for the diagnosis of AIH in patients with chronic liver disease of undetermined cause.

Nonconventional Antibodies in Diagnosis

Numerous nonconventional antibodies have also been linked to AIH and, among these, antibodies to soluble liver antigen (SLA), actin, liver cytosol type 1 (LC1), and asialoglycoprotein receptor (ASGPR) seem clinically significant and have been associated with disease severity and progression.[17]

SLA antibodies are present in 10% to 30% of white North American and northern European adults with type 1 AIH, and they have emerged as an especially promising prognostic marker. They have been shown to have a high specificity for AIH (99%), and may be present when all other serologic markers are absent.[21] They identify individuals who have severe histologic changes, invariably relapse after corticosteroid withdrawal, and have a higher frequency of liver transplantation or death from liver failure than patients without these antibodies.[22,23] A recent study found that 96% of patients with AIH with antibodies to SLA had concurrent antibodies to SSA/Ro52, and that SSA/Ro52 antibodies alone and in conjunction with SLA antibodies were independently associated with a poor prognosis.[24] The investigators hypothesized that the prognostic implications ascribed to anti-SLA may reflect their general concurrence with anti-SSA/Ro52.

Antibodies to actin are a subset of SMA that is characterized by reactivity against filamentous actin.[17] Actin antibodies that are measured by enzyme-linked immunosorbent assay methods have a sensitivity of 71% to 74% and specificity of 90% to 98% for AIH.[25,26] These performance parameters are better than those associated with SMA, determined by more labor-intensive and operator-dependent indirect immunofluorescence methods, and therefore have recently begun to replace SMA in some laboratories.[18] This shift may eventually require adaptation of the simplified diagnostic criteria. LC1 antibodies are considered a second marker of type 2 AIH, and are expressed primarily in children and young adults. They have been associated with marked liver inflammation and rapid progression to cirrhosis, and may be found in a subgroup of patients negative for ANA, SMA, and anti–LKM-1.[17,27] In addition, antibodies to ASGPR occur in most patients with both types 1 and 2 AIH (67%–88%). Their persistence or disappearance during corticosteroid therapy reflects the adequacy of treatment, and similarly their reappearance after therapy cessation is associated with disease relapse.[28] Therefore, unlike the previously discussed prognostic markers, ASGPR antibodies seem to have clinical significance when they are absent.[17]

Absence of Antibodies in Diagnosis

None of the autoantibodies mentioned earlier are a requisite for AIH, and their absence does not preclude the diagnosis. A recent comprehensive report on autoantibody-negative AIH defines the disease as meeting the IAIHG diagnostic criteria of classic AIH, but lacking the regularly measured serologic markers (ie, ANA, SMA, and anti–LKM-1).[29] The revised IAIHG scoring system can accommodate such patients if other features of AIH are sufficiently strong to counterbalance the absence of antibodies. Autoantibodies can appear and disappear throughout the course of the disease, and their absence at presentation should

neither result in misclassification as cryptogenic chronic hepatitis nor delay initiation of corticosteroids.[29] Nonconventional antibodies are not routinely tested for, but may help identify, patients with AIH in otherwise borderline cases.

MICROSCOPIC FEATURES

Although insufficient by itself, the microscopic examination of liver tissue is an essential component to the diagnosis and management of AIH.[5] In the revised IAIHG scoring system (see Table 2), histologic features compatible with AIH constitute 19% of the maximum possible score for a definite diagnosis. The absence of these features and the presence of changes incompatible with AIH reduce the score by 42%.[30] This finding shows the emphasis placed on liver biopsy interpretation, which, when analyzed for key diagnostic features, has a specificity for AIH as high as 81% and a positive predictive value of 68%.[31]

Interface hepatitis is the sine qua non of classic AIH.[5] Dense lymphocytic, often lymphoplasmacytic, infiltrates extend from the portal tracts into the lobules where they are associated with hepatocyte injury, including pyknotic necroses, ballooning degeneration, and lobular disarray (Fig. 1). Emperipolesis (penetration of intact inflammatory cells into the cytoplasm of hepatocytes) can be a helpful finding, and is one of 3 histologic features included in the simplified diagnostic criteria (see Table 3).[7] Plasma cells are often abundant in the periportal region and may extend throughout the lobule; however, 34% of patients with AIH have few or no plasma cells and this does not preclude the diagnosis (Fig. 2).[31] In our experience, a marked number of eosinophils may also be encountered (see Figs. 1B and 2B), and should not be misinterpreted as necessarily indicating drug-induced injury. Giant syncytial multinucleated hepatocytes are a nonspecific reaction to injury that can be seen in AIH (Fig. 3), but are also commonly associated with drug toxicity and viral infections, especially paramyxovirus.[32]

Panacinar hepatitis with bridging or multiacinar necrosis can develop, and signifies severe inflammation and an absolute indication for corticosteroid therapy.[30] However, the most impressive necroinflammatory lesions are typically found at the portal-lobular interface. Severe interface activity with confluent necrosis results in parenchymal collapse with regenerating hepatocytes forming rosettes around a single central canaliculus (Fig. 4).[33] This collapse can mimic fibrous bands on hematoxylin and eosin and trichrome stains,

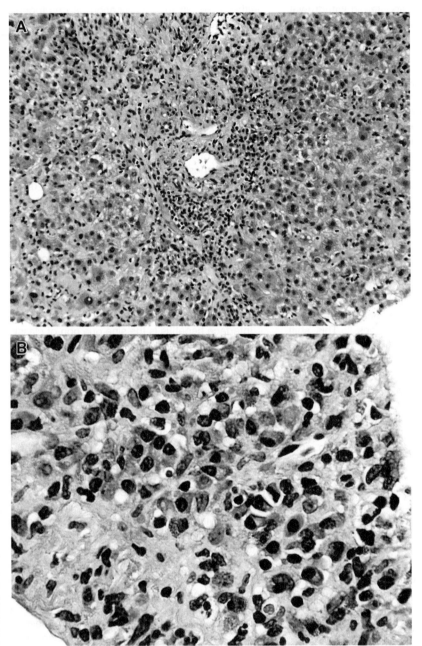

Fig. 1. (A) A portal tract expanded by a predominantly mononuclear inflammatory infiltrate that extends out circumferentially into the surrounding lobule. (B) The portal inflammatory infiltrate consists predominantly of plasma cells with many interspersed eosinophils.

and a reticulin stain may be needed for reliable differentiation (Fig. 5). In undiagnosed or untreated patients, the disease can progress to true fibrosis and ultimately cirrhosis. A recent study found that 36% of patients with AIH are cirrhotic at the time of presentation.[34] The pattern of fibrosis does not differ greatly from other forms of hepatitis and fails to provide diagnostic clues.[33]

Histologic features of cholangitis are found in up to 20% of patients who otherwise satisfy the revised scoring system criteria for AIH, and likely represent collateral damage caused by an

Fig. 1. (*C*) The inflammatory infiltrate extending
out of the portal tract
into the lobule causes damage and death of hepato-
cytes. (*D*) Marked lobular
inflammation with bal-
looned hepatocytes (*short
arrows*), acidophilic body
(*long arrow*), and macro-
phage clusters (*arrow-
heads*) cause a pattern of
lobular disarray. Asterisk
marks the central vein.

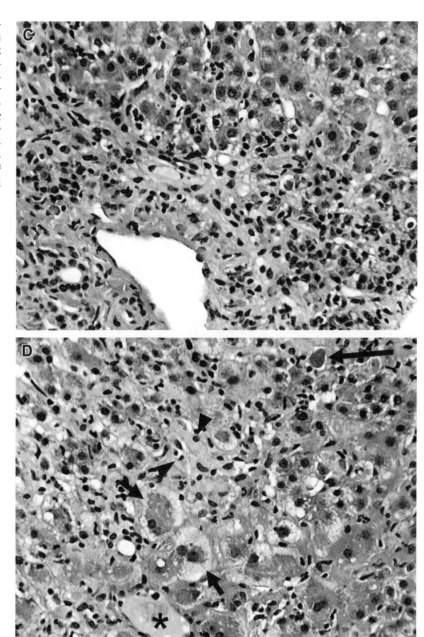

exuberant inflammatory reaction within the portal tracts (Fig. 6).[35] Ductopenia is not a feature of classic AIH. The presence of cholangitis, if not associated with a cholestatic clinical picture, is outweighed by the classic features of AIH and does not represent or evolve into a clinically significant syndrome. In a similar way, 16% of patients with AIH may show incidental steatosis.[31]

Acute and fulminant forms of AIH were recognized by the IAIHG in 1992 when they waived the requirement for 6 months of disease activity to establish the diagnosis.[5] Approximately 25% of

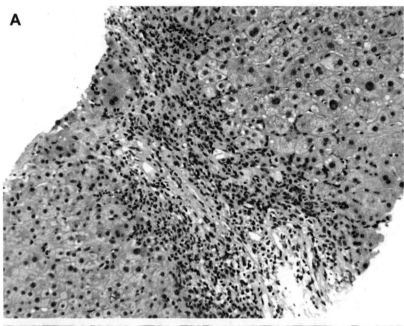

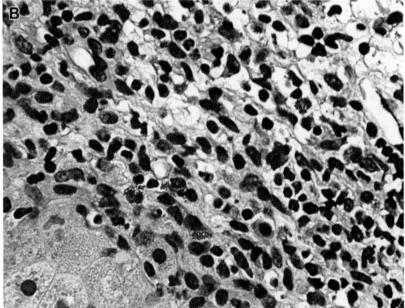

Fig. 2. (*A*) A portal tract expanded by a predominantly mononuclear inflammatory infiltrate that extends out circumferentially into the surrounding lobule. (*B*) Although scattered plasma cells are seen, the portal inflammatory infiltrate consists predominantly of lymphocytes with interspersed eosinophils.

patients have an acute onset of AIH, and rarely a fulminant presentation occurs.[16] This acute onset may represent newly developed disease[36,37] or exacerbation of a previously unrecognized chronic course.[38] The histologic patterns that characterize acute-onset AIH include a panacinar hepatitis that resembles acute viral or drug-induced hepatitis and centrilobular (zone 3) necrosis or perivenulitis that resembles an acute toxic injury (**Fig. 7**).[32] In the previously mentioned report by the Acute Liver Failure Study Group, the most common histologic feature in their cohort of patients with autoimmune

Fig. 3. AIH with lobular inflammation and damaged multinucleated hepatocytes (*arrows*).

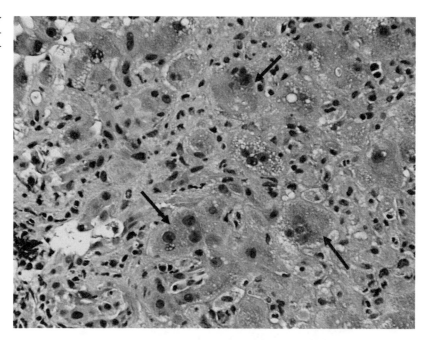

acute liver failure was central perivenulitis/necrosis,[16] which may either accompany interface activity or be the principal finding with portal tract sparing.[39] The transition from perivenular hepatitis to interface hepatitis has been shown in successive biopsies from patients with acute-onset AIH,[40] and thus the perivenular pattern may reflect an early stage of illness that is not present in later biopsy specimens.[39] In patients who are experiencing an acute exacerbation of chronic indolent disease, histologic features of chronicity, including fibrous septa or cirrhosis, may be seen.[41]

Fig. 4. AIH with hepatocytes forming rosettes (*arrows*) around a central lumen containing bile.

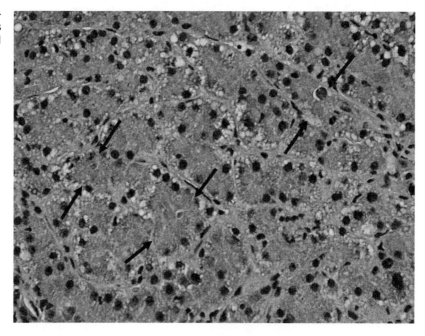

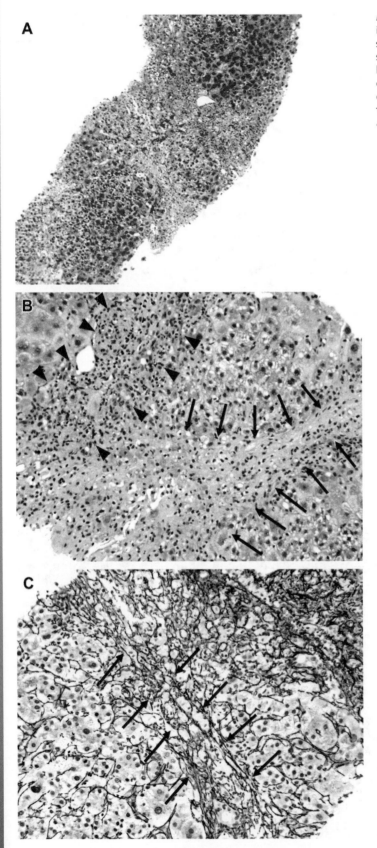

Fig. 5. (*A*) Bridging necrosis appearing as fibrous bands on trichrome stain. (*B*) On hematoxylin and eosin staining, these apparent fibrous bands correspond with bridging necrosis (*arrows*) and a longitudinally cut portal tract (*arrowheads*). (*C*) Reticulin stain highlights the bridging area of collapse (*arrows*).

Fig. 6. A bile duct (*arrows*) entrapped within the inflammatory infiltrate of AIH shows evidence of epithelial damage.

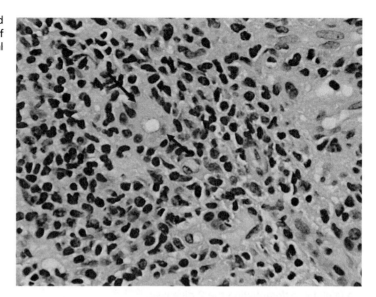

Fig. 7. (*A*) Central perivenulitis characterized by inflammation and cell loss around the central vein (*asterisk*). Arrows point to a portal tract; periportal inflammation and damage is disproportionately less than the amount of perivenular damage. The lobular parenchyma between these two structures shows inflammation and hepatocyte damage. (*B*) Inflammation consisting of lymphocytes and plasma cells with interspersed eosinophils is present around the central vein (*asterisk*) causing hepatocyte damage and cell loss.

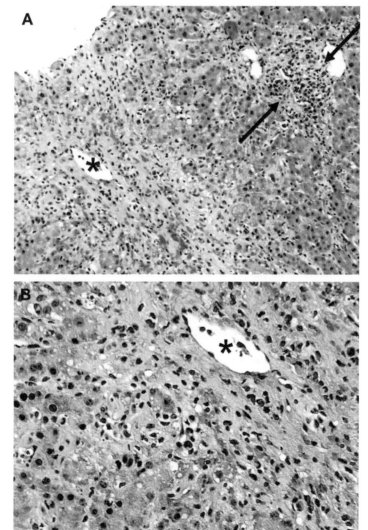

DIFFERENTIAL DIAGNOSIS

The histopathologic features of AIH comprise a constellation of findings, many of which are common to various other chronic liver disorders, such as chronic viral hepatitis, drug-induced liver injury (DILI), Wilson disease, primary biliary cirrhosis (PBC), and primary sclerosing cholangitis (PSC). These diseases encompass the differential diagnoses of AIH; nevertheless, there are several characteristic histologic findings, and combinations thereof, that can aid the pathologist in arriving at the correct diagnosis.

Chronic Hepatitis C Versus AIH

Chronic hepatitis C and AIH have significant overlapping morphologies; however, multiple studies have concluded that certain histologic features are useful in differentiating the 2 diseases.[30,31,42]

Features more commonly observed in chronic hepatitis C are:

- Steatosis (72% vs 19%)
- Portal tract lymphoid follicles (49% vs 10%)

Conversely, features more commonly seen in AIH are[42]:

- Severe lobular inflammation and necrosis (76% vs 38%)
- Severe interface hepatitis (81% vs 10%)
- Multinucleated giant hepatocytes (29% vs 6%)
- Broad areas of parenchymal collapse (76% vs 6%)

Also:

- The interface activity of chronic hepatitis C tends to be patchy and focal, whereas this tends to be more uniform in AIH.
- Confluent and bridging necrosis are predominantly seen in AIH, whereas spotty necrosis is more commonly encountered in chronic hepatitis C.[42]
- The greater degree of necrosis in AIH may explain the higher percentage of patients with cirrhosis at an earlier follow-up time, compared with patients with chronic hepatitis C.[42]
- Moderate to severe portal plasma cell infiltration is not specific for AIH, but its presence does support the diagnosis, and it is more common in this condition (66%) than in chronic hepatitis C (21%).[31]

Although bile duct damage and bile duct loss have been occasionally reported to be more common in chronic hepatitis C than in AIH (91% vs 40% and 91% vs 20% respectively), this high incidence of bile duct damage and loss cannot be corroborated by us.

DILI Versus AIH

DILI can mimic almost any pattern of injury observed with primary liver diseases. When causing a chronic or acute hepatitic pattern, differentiating DILI from AIH can be challenging and often impossible. Suzuki and colleagues[43] recently performed a blinded, standardized histologic evaluation to assess the usefulness of liver biopsy in discriminating DILI from idiopathic AIH. They concluded that, although there is significant morphologic overlap between the two diseases (ie, interface hepatitis, focal necrosis, and portal inflammation were present in all evaluated cases), pathologists can use a combination of features to suggest the correct diagnosis, even in the absence of clinical information. They found that more severe portal inflammation (Ishak score ≥2), prominent portal plasma cells, rosette formation, and higher necrosis and fibrosis scores all favored a diagnosis of AIH, whereas portal neutrophils, prominent intra-acinar lymphocytes, and hepatocellular and canalicular cholestasis were more prevalent in DILI. Prominent portal and intra-acinar eosinophils were more common in cases of AIH than DILI.

Drug-Induced Autoimmune Hepatitis Versus AIH

Drug-induced AIH (DIAIH) is a specific subtype of DILI, and has been found to be caused by one of 2 drugs (minocycline or nitrofurantoin) in 90% of cases.[44] DIAIH is almost a complete mimic of idiopathic AIH, showing interface and lobular hepatitis with portal infiltrates of lymphocytes, plasma cells, and eosinophils, and a similar incidence of ANA and SMA seropositivity.[43,44] Centrilobular zone 3 necrosis may also be seen and resembles an acute-onset picture of idiopathic AIH. However, cirrhosis was not observed in any of the patients with DIAIH in 2 histologic studies, but was present in 15% to 21% of patients with idiopathic AIH.[43,44] Apart from this isolated feature, idiopathic AIH and DIAIH seem to be histologically identical, and in the study by Suzuki and colleagues[43] the complete agreement rate among pathologists was just 28.6% for the diagnosis of DIAIH and 46% for idiopathic AIH.[43] In more than 80% of patients with idiopathic AIH there is relapse within 1 year in the absence of adequate immunosuppression, whereas, in patients with DIAIH, there is no relapse.[45] This clinical characteristic is probably the most reliable feature for identifying DIAIH.

Wilson Disease Versus AIH

Like AIH, Wilson disease may present as an acute, fulminant, or chronic hepatic disease. With a fulminant presentation, differentiating between Wilson disease and AIH is critical, because some patients with fulminant-onset AIH may be salvaged with medical therapy, whereas patients with fulminant-onset Wilson disease need prompt liver transplantation to survive.[46] The two diseases share significant histologic features, including interface hepatitis with lobular inflammation, ballooning degeneration, and single-cell necrosis. Irrespective of the initial symptoms, almost all patients with Wilson disease have some evidence of cirrhosis on liver biopsy, the absence of which weakens the diagnosis.[46] Helpful histologic clues that are commonly observed in Wilson disease but not in AIH include moderate to marked steatosis, periportal glycogenated nuclei, Mallory bodies in periportal hepatocytes, and moderate to marked copper storage.[47] However, histochemical stains for copper (rhodamine, rubeanic acid), and copper-binding protein (orcein) are often unreliable, particularly in early stages of the disease, and negative staining does not preclude the diagnosis of Wilson disease.[48]

PBC Versus AIH

The diagnosis of PBC is usually straightforward based on clinical, laboratory, and serologic findings; however, liver biopsy is useful in atypical cases and in establishing the diagnosis of antimitochondrial antibody (AMA)-negative PBC.[49] Histologic findings that help distinguish PBC from AIH include bile duct destruction with granuloma formation (florid duct lesion), bile duct loss, cholate stasis, and copper accumulation.[32] Lymphocytic infiltration of bile ducts and ductular proliferation are nonspecific features that can be seen in both PBC and AIH. Lobular disarray and regenerative rosette formation are uncommon in PBC, and more strongly indicate a hepatocytic pattern of injury.[32] Discrimination of AIH from stage 2 PBC may be impossible by histology alone, if the lymphoplasmacytic portal inflammation and interface hepatitis are not accompanied by diffuse lobular hepatitis (AIH) or ductopenia or granulomas (PBC).[32] Immunohistochemical stains for IgG and immunoglobulin M (IgM) have been shown to be useful in distinguishing AIH from PBC.[50–52] Plasmacytic infiltrates expressing predominantly IgM are characteristic of PBC, whereas the plasma cells in AIH primarily stain for IgG. In one study, an IgM/IgG ratio of greater than 1 accurately distinguished PBC from AIH in 91% of cases.[51]

PSC Versus AIH

The histologic findings in PSC are variable and often nonspecific. The pathognomonic bile duct lesion is an obliterative fibrous cholangitis with periductal fibrosis or so-called onion skinning. When identified, this feature is virtually diagnostic of PSC; however, it is found in less than 40% of biopsy specimens.[32] Additional features commonly seen in PSC but not in AIH include ductopenia, neutrophilic portal infiltrates, cholate stasis, and copper accumulation.[30] Similar to PBC, stage 2 PSC can closely mimic AIH; unlike PBC, PSC seems to have the same IgG-predominate plasma cell staining pattern as AIH.[51]

ΔΔ   ***Differential Diagnosis*** OF AIH

AIH Versus	Helpful Distinguishing Features
Chronic viral hepatitis	Less severe interface activity and lobular inflammation/necrosis More frequent bile duct injury, steatosis, and portal tract lymphoid follicles Less prominent plasma cell infiltration
DILI	Less severe portal inflammation, necrosis, and fibrosis Portal neutrophils and hepatocellular/canalicular cholestasis Less prominent plasma cell infiltration
Wilson disease	Moderate to marked steatosis, glycogenated nuclei, Mallory bodies in periportal hepatocytes, and increased copper storage Greater frequency of cirrhosis at presentation
PBC	Bile duct destruction, ductopenia, granulomas, cholate stasis, copper accumulation Immunohistochemical stain showing IgM-predominate plasma cells (vs IgG-predominate plasma cells in AIH)
PSC	Obliterative fibrous cholangitis with periductal onion-skinning fibrosis Ductopenia, neutrophilic portal infiltrates, cholate stasis, copper accumulation

PROGNOSIS

Information on the natural history of AIH derived from experience before the use of immunosuppression suggests that as many as 40% of patients, if left untreated, would die within 6 months of diagnosis.[1] Immunosuppression therapy has improved survival, and treatment is effective in suppressing AIH in up to 80% of patients within 3 years.[53] Ten-year survival rates are generally promising, ranging from approximately 85% to 95%[3,34,54]; however, a recent large-cohort study reported a 20-year survival rate of only 48%,[34] suggesting that the disease process may be accelerated in the second decade. Factors associated with a poor outcome include cirrhosis, liver decompensation at presentation, delayed treatment response, and a high relapse rate.[34,53] As with other causes of cirrhosis, the development of hepatocellular carcinoma (HCC) has been observed in patients with AIH. A recent study determined that the risk of developing HCC in patients with AIH with cirrhosis is 1% to 1.9% per year.[55] This rate is similar to that seen in patients with cirrhosis secondary to hepatitis C, hepatitis B, and alcohol-related liver disease. For patients who progress to liver failure, liver transplantation may be considered, which has 5-year survival rates of approximately 75%.[56] Recurrence rates of AIH in the allograft have varied from 12% to 50%.[56]

Histologic findings can also provide important prognostic information. At presentation, a diagnosis of interface hepatitis is associated with a 17% risk of progression to cirrhosis, whereas bridging necrosis progresses to cirrhosis in 82% of cases.[32] Liver biopsy performed before drug withdrawal is the only way to confirm disease remission (defined as the absence of interface hepatitis) and histologic features can help predict the likelihood of subsequent clinical relapse. Reversion of the liver architecture to normal is associated with a 20% incidence of relapse; presence of portal inflammation only is associated with a 50% incidence of relapse; presence of interface hepatitis is associated with an 80% incidence of relapse; and progression to cirrhosis is nearly always associated with relapse.[32] Histologic features that predict a high probability of relapse must be recognized by the pathologist so that premature cessation of therapy can be avoided.

OVERLAP SYNDROMES

AIH has 2 major variant phenotypes in which the clinical, laboratory, and histologic features of classic disease are combined with those of PBC or PSC. These so-called overlap syndromes lack established diagnostic criteria and pathogenic mechanisms, and their clinical significance primarily relates to management strategies.[49] The overlap syndromes may reflect concurrent or sequential manifestations of 2 separate diseases, distinct entities on their own, or primary disorders presenting with atypical characteristics also seen in other disorders; most investigators support the theory of primary disorders presenting with atypical characteristics also seen in other disorders. A recent position statement by the IAIHG recommends that patients with autoimmune liver disease be categorized according to their predominating features as AIH, PBC, or PSC, and that overlapping features not be considered distinct diagnostic entities.[49] The prevalence of the overlap syndromes is difficult to determine because of the lack of standardized criteria and variations in patient populations between studies. Nevertheless, the frequency of the overlap syndromes with PBC and PSC in patients originally diagnosed as having AIH ranges from 7% to 13% and 6% to 11%, respectively.[57]

Diagnostic criteria, referred to as the Paris criteria, have been proposed for the diagnosis of AIH-PBC overlap syndrome. Although endorsed by some medical centers, these criteria are arbitrary because of limited current knowledge regarding the pathogenesis of either AIH or PBC.[49] These criteria require the presence of at least 2 of 3 recognized hallmarks of each disease.[58]

The 3 hallmarks of AIH are:

1. Serum alanine aminotransferase concentration 5 times or greater the upper limit of normal (ULN)
2. IgG concentration greater than twice the ULN or a positive test for SMA
3. Histologic features of moderate to severe interface hepatitis

The 3 hallmarks of PBC are:

1. Serum alkaline phosphatase concentration greater than twice the ULN or gamma glutamyl transpeptidase concentration 5 times or greater the ULN
2. Positive AMA test
3. Histologic evidence of florid duct lesions

In a recent study, these criteria had a sensitivity and specificity for AIH-PBC overlap syndrome of 92% and 97%, respectively, when using clinical judgment as the gold standard for diagnosis, and they performed superiorly to both the revised original and simplified scoring systems of the IAIHG.[59] These findings support the IAIHG position statement that the AIH scoring systems were not designed, and should therefore not be used, for establishing diagnoses of overlap syndromes.[49] The histologic features of AIH-PBC overlap syndrome include a variable combination of lymphoplasmacytic infiltrates directed at biliary epithelium and hepatocytes, producing bile duct injury and loss, interface hepatitis, and parenchymal necroinflammation.[41]

The diagnosis of AIH-PSC overlap syndrome typically requires predominant features of AIH by the IAIHG diagnostic criteria, absence of AMA, and features of cholestasis, including increased alkaline phosphatase and bile duct injury or loss on histology.[57] Characteristic focal strictures and dilatations (beading) of the biliary tree by magnetic resonance cholangiography typify most cases; however, negative radiographic studies do not preclude the diagnosis, because detectable bile duct changes may emerge later in the disease course and a small-duct PSC variant has been described.[60] In pediatric patients, PSC is often associated with marked autoimmune features, including autoantibodies, increased IgG, and interface hepatitis. This overlap syndrome, termed autoimmune sclerosing cholangitis, has the same prevalence as AIH type 1 in childhood and patients respond equally well to immunosuppressant therapy.[61] In a 16-year prospective study including 55 children who presented with evidence of liver disease and circulating autoantibodies, 49% of patients had bile duct abnormalities consistent with PSC on cholangiography, and the remaining 51% were diagnosed with AIH. Of the 27 patients with PSC, 52% also satisfied the IAIHG criteria for definite AIH.[61] Thirty-five percent of the patients with PSC had no histologic biliary changes; cholangiography is therefore necessary to exclude an overlap of PSC in pediatric patients with AIH.

IMMUNOGLOBULIN G4–ASSOCIATED AIH

Immunoglobulin G4 (IgG4)–mediated diseases are being increasingly recognized and have been an area of active research. Two Japanese groups recently investigated the possible existence of a distinct subset of AIH associated with IgG4. Chung and colleagues[62] observed positive IgG4 immunostaining in 9 of 26 (34.6%) patients with AIH, with a positive cutoff value of more than 5 IgG4+ plasma cells per high-power field (hpf). In contrast, none of their PBC (n = 10), PSC (n = 3), or hepatitis C virus (n = 20) cases stained positive for IgG4. The patients with IgG4-associated AIH showed more severe portal inflammation, with greater plasma cell infiltration, and higher total serum IgG levels than the patients with IgG4-nonassociated AIH. However, none of the patients with IgG4-

associated AIH had increased serum IgG4 levels, which is generally accepted as one of the defining features of IgG4-related diseases.[63] These patients also showed a dramatic and sustained response to prednisolone, with no patients experiencing relapse, compared with a 37.5% relapse rate in patients with IgG4 nonassociated AIH. The investigators concluded that IgG4 immunostaining may have prognostic usefulness in patients with AIH by identifying a subpopulation that shows a marked response to steroid therapy. Further studies using larger patient groups are needed to confirm these findings.

A second set of investigators (Umemura and colleagues[64]) applied more stringent criteria to the diagnosis of IgG4-associated AIH, requiring greater than 10 IgG4+ plasma cells per hpf, an increased serum IgG4 level ($\geq$135 mg/dL), and definite AIH by the IAIHG scoring system, and found the prevalence to be only 3.3% (2 of 60 patients). These two patients had more severe histologic changes, including marked plasma cell infiltration and giant hepatocyte and rosette formation, but lack of bile duct damage, and again a favorable response to steroid treatment.

Patients with autoimmune pancreatitis often have various extrapancreatic lesions that share common histopathologic findings, including IgG4+ plasma cell infiltrates. It has been proposed that autoimmune pancreatitis is not simply a pancreatitis, but a pancreatic manifestation of a larger systemic syndrome termed IgG4-related

Pitfalls
IN AIH

! Plasma cells are common in AIH, but their absence does not preclude the diagnosis. Eosinophils are also frequently seen and do not necessarily indicate drug-induced injury.

! Parenchymal collapse caused by confluent necrosis can mimic fibrous bands and may require a reticulin stain for differentiation.

! Up to 20% of patients who otherwise satisfy diagnostic criteria for AIH may show coincidental bile duct injury or loss, which, in the absence of a cholestatic clinical picture, are clinically insignificant changes and should not be misdiagnosed as an overlap syndrome.

! The histologic features of acute-onset AIH may closely resemble acute viral hepatitis, DILI, or Wilson disease and must be interpreted in light of correlating clinical information.

sclerosing disease.[65] Umemura and colleagues[66] reported that almost all patients with autoimmune pancreatitis have coexistent liver dysfunction with histologic changes such as interface and lobular hepatitis and abundant IgG4+ plasma cells, which they termed IgG4 hepatopathy. An important question arising from the two studies discussed earlier is whether IgG4-associated AIH is a hepatic manifestation of autoimmune pancreatitis/IgG4-related sclerosing disease, or a subtype of classic AIH. In support of the latter, none of the patients with IgG4-associated AIH had pancreatic enlargement or bile duct abnormalities by imaging, or any other lesions of IgG4-related sclerosing disease.[62,64] Future studies are needed to elucidate the true nature of these IgG4-associated AIH cases.

REFERENCES

1. Gossard AA, Lindor KD. Autoimmune hepatitis: a review. J Gastroenterol 2012;47:498–503.
2. Ngu JH, Bechly K, Chapman BA, et al. Population-based epidemiology study of autoimmune hepatitis: a disease of older women? J Gastroenterol Hepatol 2010;25:1681–6.
3. Kanzler S, Lohr H, Gerken G, et al. Long-term management and prognosis of autoimmune hepatitis (AIH): a single center experience. Z Gastroenterol 2001;39:339–41, 344–8.
4. Lohse AW, Wiegard C. Diagnostic criteria for autoimmune hepatitis. Best Pract Res Clin Gastroenterol 2011;25:665–71.
5. Alvarez F, Berg PA, Bianchi FB, et al. International Autoimmune Hepatitis Group Report: review of criteria for diagnosis of autoimmune hepatitis. J Hepatol 1999;31:929–38.
6. Manns MP, Czaja AJ, Gorham JD, et al. Diagnosis and management of autoimmune hepatitis. Hepatology 2010;51:2193–213.
7. Hennes EM, Zeniya M, Czaja AJ, et al. Simplified criteria for the diagnosis of autoimmune hepatitis. Hepatology 2008;48:169–76.
8. Czaja AJ. Performance parameters of the diagnostic scoring systems for autoimmune hepatitis. Hepatology 2008;48:1540–8.
9. Muratori P, Granito A, Pappas G, et al. Validation of simplified diagnostic criteria for autoimmune hepatitis in Italian patients. Hepatology 2009;49:1782–3 [author reply: 3].
10. Gatselis NK, Zachou K, Papamichalis P, et al. Comparison of simplified score with the revised original score for the diagnosis of autoimmune hepatitis: a new or a complementary diagnostic score? Dig Liver Dis 2010;42:807–12.
11. Qiu D, Wang Q, Wang H, et al. Validation of the simplified criteria for diagnosis of autoimmune hepatitis in Chinese patients. J Hepatol 2011;54:340–7.
12. Fujiwara K, Yasui S, Tawada A, et al. Diagnostic value and utility of the simplified International Autoimmune Hepatitis Group criteria in acute-onset autoimmune hepatitis. Liver Int 2011;31:1013–20.
13. Yeoman AD, Westbrook RH, Al-Chalabi T, et al. Diagnostic value and utility of the simplified International Autoimmune Hepatitis Group (IAIHG) criteria in acute and chronic liver disease. Hepatology 2009;50:538–45.
14. Mileti E, Rosenthal P, Peters MG. Validation and modification of simplified diagnostic criteria for autoimmune hepatitis in children. Clin Gastroenterol Hepatol 2012;10:417–421.e1–2.
15. Miyake Y, Iwasaki Y, Kobashi H, et al. Clinical features of autoimmune hepatitis diagnosed based on simplified criteria of the International Autoimmune Hepatitis Group. Dig Liver Dis 2010;42:210–5.
16. Stravitz RT, Lefkowitch JH, Fontana RJ, et al. Autoimmune acute liver failure: proposed clinical and histological criteria. Hepatology 2011;53:517–26.
17. Czaja AJ. Autoantibodies as prognostic markers in autoimmune liver disease. Dig Dis Sci 2010;55:2144–61.
18. Krawitt EL. Discrimination of autoimmune hepatitis: autoantibody typing and beyond. J Gastroenterol 2011;46(Suppl 1):39–41.
19. Mehendiratta V, Mitroo P, Bombonati A, et al. Serologic markers do not predict histologic severity or response to treatment in patients with autoimmune hepatitis. Clin Gastroenterol Hepatol 2009;7:98–103.
20. Czaja AJ. Performance parameters of the conventional serological markers for autoimmune hepatitis. Dig Dis Sci 2011;56:545–54.
21. Baeres M, Herkel J, Czaja AJ, et al. Establishment of standardised SLA/LP immunoassays: specificity for autoimmune hepatitis, worldwide occurrence, and clinical characteristics. Gut 2002;51:259–64.
22. Ma Y, Okamoto M, Thomas MG, et al. Antibodies to conformational epitopes of soluble liver antigen define a severe form of autoimmune liver disease. Hepatology 2002;35:658–64.
23. Czaja AJ, Donaldson PT, Lohse AW. Antibodies to soluble liver antigen/liver pancreas and HLA risk factors for type 1 autoimmune hepatitis. Am J Gastroenterol 2002;97:413–9.
24. Montano-Loza AJ, Shums Z, Norman GL, et al. Prognostic implications of antibodies to Ro/SSA and soluble liver antigen in type 1 autoimmune hepatitis. Liver Int 2012;32:85–92.
25. Aubert V, Pisler IG, Spertini F. Improved diagnoses of autoimmune hepatitis using an anti-actin ELISA. J Clin Lab Anal 2008;22:340–5.
26. Frenzel C, Herkel J, Luth S, et al. Evaluation of F-actin ELISA for the diagnosis of autoimmune hepatitis. Am J Gastroenterol 2006;101:2731–6.
27. Bridoux-Henno L, Maggiore G, Johanet C, et al. Features and outcome of autoimmune hepatitis

type 2 presenting with isolated positivity for anti-liver cytosol antibody. Clin Gastroenterol Hepatol 2004;2:825–30.

28. Hausdorf G, Roggenbuck D, Feist E, et al. Autoantibodies to asialoglycoprotein receptor (ASGPR) measured by a novel ELISA–revival of a disease-activity marker in autoimmune hepatitis. Clin Chim Acta 2009;408:19–24.

29. Czaja AJ. Autoantibody-negative autoimmune hepatitis. Dig Dis Sci 2012;57:610–24.

30. Carpenter HA, Czaja AJ. The role of histologic evaluation in the diagnosis and management of autoimmune hepatitis and its variants. Clin Liver Dis 2002; 6:685–705.

31. Czaja AJ, Carpenter HA. Sensitivity, specificity, and predictability of biopsy interpretations in chronic hepatitis. Gastroenterology 1993;105:1824–32.

32. Czaja AJ, Carpenter HA. Autoimmune hepatitis. In: Burt AD, Portmann BC, Ferrell LD, editors. MacSween's pathology of the liver. 5th edition. Edinburgh (Scotland): Churchill Livingstone; 2007. p. 493–515.

33. Meyer zum Buschenfelde KH, Dienes HP. Autoimmune hepatitis. Definition–classification–histopathology–immunopathogenesis. Virchows Arch 1996; 429:1–12.

34. Hoeroldt B, McFarlane E, Dube A, et al. Long-term outcomes of patients with autoimmune hepatitis managed at a nontransplant center. Gastroenterology 2011;140:1980–9.

35. Czaja AJ, Carpenter HA. Autoimmune hepatitis with incidental histologic features of bile duct injury. Hepatology 2001;34:659–65.

36. Kessler WR, Cummings OW, Eckert G, et al. Fulminant hepatic failure as the initial presentation of acute autoimmune hepatitis. Clin Gastroenterol Hepatol 2004;2:625–31.

37. Okano N, Yamamoto K, Sakaguchi K, et al. Clinicopathological features of acute-onset autoimmune hepatitis. Hepatol Res 2003;25:263–70.

38. Burgart LJ, Batts KP, Ludwig J, et al. Recent-onset autoimmune hepatitis. Biopsy findings and clinical correlations. Am J Surg Pathol 1995;19: 699–708.

39. Hofer H, Oesterreicher C, Wrba F, et al. Centrilobular necrosis in autoimmune hepatitis: a histological feature associated with acute clinical presentation. J Clin Pathol 2006;59:246–9.

40. Singh R, Nair S, Farr G, et al. Acute autoimmune hepatitis presenting with centrizonal liver disease: case report and review of the literature. Am J Gastroenterol 2002;97:2670–3.

41. Guindi M. Histology of autoimmune hepatitis and its variants. Clin Liver Dis 2010;14:577–90.

42. Bach N, Thung SN, Schaffner F. The histological features of chronic hepatitis C and autoimmune chronic hepatitis: a comparative analysis. Hepatology 1992;15:572–7.

43. Suzuki A, Brunt EM, Kleiner DE, et al. The use of liver biopsy evaluation in discrimination of idiopathic autoimmune hepatitis versus drug-induced liver injury. Hepatology 2011;54:931–9.

44. Bjornsson E, Talwalkar J, Treeprasertsuk S, et al. Drug-induced autoimmune hepatitis: clinical characteristics and prognosis. Hepatology 2010;51: 2040–8.

45. Aithal GP, Watkins PB, Andrade RJ, et al. Case definition and phenotype standardization in drug-induced liver injury. Clin Pharmacol Ther 2011;89: 806–15.

46. Santos RG, Alissa F, Reyes J, et al. Fulminant hepatic failure: Wilson's disease or autoimmune hepatitis? Implications for transplantation. Pediatr Transplant 2005;9:112–6.

47. Portmann BC, Thompson RJ, Eve AR, et al. Genetic and metabolic liver disease. In: Burt AD, Portmann BC, Ferrell LD, editors. MacSween's pathology of the liver. 5th edition. Edinburgh (Scotland): Churchill Livingstone; 2007. p. 249–54.

48. Pilloni L, Lecca S, Van Eyken P, et al. Value of histochemical stains for copper in the diagnosis of Wilson's disease. Histopathology 1998;33:28–33.

49. Boberg KM, Chapman RW, Hirschfield GM, et al. Overlap syndromes: the International Autoimmune Hepatitis Group (IAIHG) position statement on a controversial issue. J Hepatol 2011;54:374–85.

50. Daniels JA, Torbenson M, Anders RA, et al. Immunostaining of plasma cells in primary biliary cirrhosis. Am J Clin Pathol 2009;131:243–9.

51. Moreira RK, Revetta F, Koehler E, et al. Diagnostic utility of IgG and IgM immunohistochemistry in autoimmune liver disease. World J Gastroenterol 2010;16:453–7.

52. Cabibi D, Tarantino G, Barbaria F, et al. Intrahepatic IgG/IgM plasma cells ratio helps in classifying autoimmune liver diseases. Dig Liver Dis 2010;42: 585–92.

53. Czaja AJ. Rapidity of treatment response and outcome in type 1 autoimmune hepatitis. J Hepatol 2009;51:161–7.

54. Malekzadeh Z, Haghazali S, Sepanlou SG, et al. Clinical features and long term outcome of 102 treated autoimmune hepatitis patients. Hepat Mon 2012;12:92–9.

55. Wong RJ, Gish R, Frederick T, et al. Development of hepatocellular carcinoma in autoimmune hepatitis patients: a case series. Dig Dis Sci 2011;56: 578–85.

56. Ilyas JA, O'Mahony CA, Vierling JM. Liver transplantation in autoimmune liver diseases. Best Pract Res Clin Gastroenterol 2011;25:765–82.

57. Czaja AJ. The Overlap syndromes of autoimmune hepatitis. Dig Dis Sci 2013;58(2):326–43.

58. Chazouilleres O, Wendum D, Serfaty L, et al. Primary biliary cirrhosis-autoimmune hepatitis overlap

syndrome: clinical features and response to therapy. Hepatology 1998;28:296–301.

59. Kuiper EM, Zondervan PE, van Buuren HR. Paris criteria are effective in diagnosis of primary biliary cirrhosis and autoimmune hepatitis overlap syndrome. Clin Gastroenterol Hepatol 2010;8: 530–4.

60. Olsson R, Glaumann H, Almer S, et al. High prevalence of small duct primary sclerosing cholangitis among patients with overlapping autoimmune hepatitis and primary sclerosing cholangitis. Eur J Intern Med 2009;20:190–6.

61. Gregorio GV, Portmann B, Karani J, et al. Autoimmune hepatitis/sclerosing cholangitis overlap syndrome in childhood: a 16-year prospective study. Hepatology 2001;33:544–53.

62. Chung H, Watanabe T, Kudo M, et al. Identification and characterization of IgG4-associated autoimmune hepatitis. Liver Int 2010;30:222–31.

63. Cheuk W, Chan JK. IgG4-related sclerosing disease: a critical appraisal of an evolving clinicopathologic entity. Adv Anat Pathol 2010;17:303–32.

64. Umemura T, Zen Y, Hamano H, et al. Clinical significance of immunoglobulin G4-associated autoimmune hepatitis. J Gastroenterol 2011;46(Suppl 1):48–55.

65. Kamisawa T, Okamoto A. Autoimmune pancreatitis: proposal of IgG4-related sclerosing disease. J Gastroenterol 2006;41:613–25.

66. Umemura T, Zen Y, Hamano H, et al. Immunoglobin G4-hepatopathy: association of immunoglobin G4-bearing plasma cells in liver with autoimmune pancreatitis. Hepatology 2007;46:463–71.

Liver Transplant Pathology
Review of Challenging Diagnostic Situations

Bita V. Naini, MD[a],*, Charles R. Lassman, MD, PhD[b]

KEYWORDS

- Acute cellular rejection • Late acute rejection • Chronic rejection • Plasma cell hepatitis
- Idiopathic posttransplant chronic hepatitis • Fibrosing cholestatic hepatitis • CMV hepatitis
- EBV hepatitis • Hepatitis E • Acute antibody-mediated rejection

ABSTRACT

Histopathologic assessment of allograft liver biopsies has an important role in managing patients who have undergone liver transplantation. In this review, several topics are discussed that create diagnostic problems in transplant pathology, with emphasis on pathologic features and differential diagnosis. The topics discussed are acute cellular rejection, late acute rejection (centrizonal/parenchymal rejection), chronic rejection, plasma cell hepatitis, idiopathic posttransplant chronic hepatitis, fibrosing cholestatic hepatitis, selected viral infections (cytomegalovirus, Epstein-Barr virus, and hepatitis E), and acute antibody-mediated rejection.

OVERVIEW

Orthotopic liver transplantation (OLT) is the current gold standard of care in patients with end-stage liver disease, acute liver failure, and selected primary malignancies. Many of the common posttransplant complications cannot be differentiated from each other clinically and biochemically. In addition, more than 1 factor might be contributing to graft dysfunction. Hence, histopathologic assessment of allograft liver biopsies has an important role in differential diagnosis of posttransplant complications, identifying the cause of graft damage, and subsequently initiating appropriate therapeutic intervention. On the other hand, because many of these complications share similar histopathologic findings, it is necessary for

pathologists to incorporate all pertinent clinical, laboratory, and imaging findings with their histopathologic assessment. In this review, some specific areas are addressed that create diagnostic problems in liver transplant pathology and approaches are suggested for resolving these diagnostic dilemmas.

ACUTE CELLULAR REJECTION

Acute cellular rejection (ACR) is the most common complication in the early posttransplant period and the most common type of rejection. Although it is generally treatable and rarely affects graft function, about 10% of patients with ACR develop chronic rejection (CR), which can lead to graft failure. Most ACR cases occur between 5 and 30 days after transplant, but ACR may occur as early as 2 days or as late as many months after transplantation.[1,2] Laboratory findings lack specificity, and thus histopathologic assessment is still the gold standard for diagnosis.

The histopathologic features of ACR have been defined as a triad of:

1. Mixed portal inflammation
2. Bile duct inflammation/damage
3. Portal or central vein endotheliitis

The minimum diagnostic criteria for ACR are generally accepted as the presence of at least 2 of the aforementioned features.[1–5] However, because these features may vary considerably in different areas of the graft, it is recommended to examine a minimum of 5 portal tracts and at least

[a] Department of Pathology and Laboratory Medicine, David Geffen School of Medicine at UCLA, 10833 Le Conte Avenue, 1P-172 CHS, Los Angeles, CA 90095-1732, USA; [b] Department of Pathology and Laboratory Medicine, David Geffen School of Medicine at UCLA, 10833 Le Conte Ave, 13-145 CHS, Los Angeles, CA 90095-1732, USA
* Corresponding author.
E-mail address: bnaini@mednet.ucla.edu

Surgical Pathology 6 (2013) 277–293
http://dx.doi.org/10.1016/j.path.2013.03.004

2 sections at different levels when evaluating allograft core biopsies for ACR.[2]

The portal inflammatory infiltrate in ACR is mixed and consists predominantly of lymphocytes, including large activated immunoblasts with large nuclei, prominent nucleoli, and abundant basophilic cytoplasm. Other inflammatory cells include eosinophils, plasma cells, macrophages, and occasional neutrophils (**Fig. 1**A). The presence of conspicuous portal eosinophils is a helpful histologic clue to the diagnosis of ACR.[6] The portal infiltrates range from mild to severe, and can involve few to all sampled portal tracts. In most mild cases of ACR, the inflammatory infiltrate is limited to the portal tracts. The presence of prominent interface hepatitis indicates either a more severe form of ACR, a late form of ACR (see later discussion), or another concomitant cause of hepatitis.

Bile duct inflammation/damage is characterized by lymphocytic infiltration of the duct epithelium, typically associated with epithelial cell injury. This

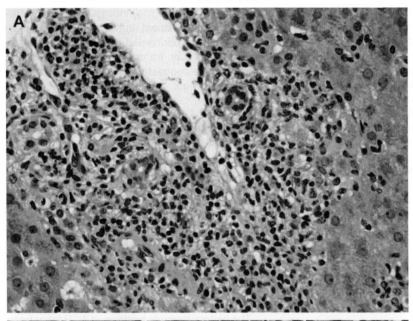

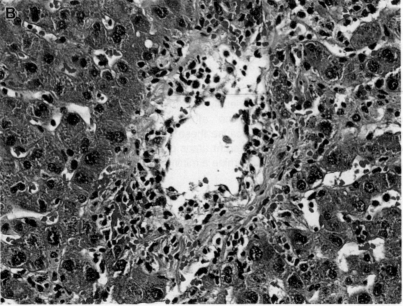

Fig. 1. ACR. (*A*) There is mixed portal inflammatory infiltrate (predominantly lymphocytic with admixed eosinophils) in addition to bile duct injury and portal vein endotheliitis. Bile duct injury is shown as lymphocytic infiltration of the duct epithelium accompanied by nuclear enlargement, overlapping, and loss of polarity. (*B*) Central vein endotheliitis in a case of moderate acute rejection. The prominent subendothelial lymphocytic infiltrate is lifting up and disrupting the overlying endothelium.

injury is manifested as loss of nuclear polarity caused by variable nuclear enlargement, overlapping nuclei, pleomorphism, apoptosis, cytoplasmic vacuolization, and luminal disruption. Bile ductular reaction is usually insignificant (see **Fig. 1A**).

Endotheliitis is the most specific diagnostic feature of ACR. Endotheliitis most commonly involves portal veins, but central veins are also frequently involved in more severe cases. Endotheliitis is characterized by subendothelial lymphocytic infiltrates that lift up and detach the overlying endothelium from the basement membrane. Endothelial cells may be swollen and plump (see **Fig. 1B**).

In recent years, there has been increasing awareness of a larger spectrum of histologic changes that may occur in acute rejection, especially later in the posttransplant course (see later discussion).

LATE ACUTE REJECTION (CENTRIZONAL/ PARENCHYMAL REJECTION)

Late acute rejection (LAR) refers to a form of cellular rejection that occurs several months after transplantation and may show different histologic features as compared to typical ACR described earlier. Patients with LAR are more likely to be resistant to increased immunosuppression and may have a higher risk for CR, fibrosis, and graft loss.[7–12] This form of rejection has also been variously named centrizonal/parenchymal rejection, hepatitic variant of ACR, or atypical rejection.

Pathology of LAR

Pathologically, LAR usually resembles chronic hepatitis with interface and lobular activity (with or without plasma cell rich infiltrates) and typically with zone 3 inflammation (ie, central perivenulitis [CPV]). CPV is characterized by an inflammatory infiltrate surrounding the central veins, which may or may not be associated with centrilobular hepatocyte injury, dropout, and necrosis (**Fig. 2**). CPV may be seen in isolation or in association with portal-based features of ACR and may or may not be accompanied by central vein endotheliitis.[11,13,14] In the presence of characteristic portal changes of rejection, CPV is a sign of severe ACR, whereas isolated CPV is a histologic finding that may be seen in LAR.[15–18] Compared with typical ACR, LAR is also less likely to have blastic lymphocytes, portal eosinophils, bile duct damage, and endotheliitis.

Differential Diagnosis in LAR

A major differential diagnosis of acute rejection, particularly LAR, is viral hepatitis, especially recurrent hepatitis C virus (HCV). HCV infection is the most common indication for OLT in the United States, and recurrent hepatitis C is nearly universal. Reinfection by hepatitis C occurs during allograft reperfusion, and pretransplant viral titers are reached in about 72 hours.[19] Therefore, the

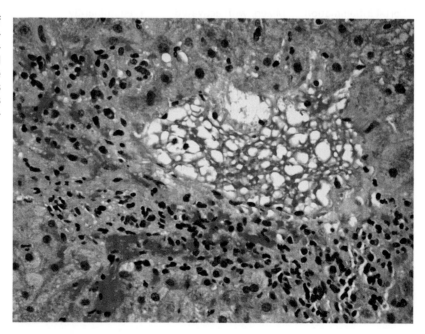

Fig. 2. CPV in a case of LAR. An inflammatory infiltrate surrounds a central vein with associated perivenular hepatocyte necrosis/dropout. In this case, the portal tracts did not show typical features of acute rejection.

diagnostic dilemma in posttransplant biopsies is usually not recurrent HCV versus ACR, but rather recurrent HCV with or without concomitant ACR.

Another important differential diagnosis of ACR is recurrent primary biliary cirrhosis (PBC). Recurrence of PBC in liver allografts is now well accepted.[20] The more characteristic and diagnostic features of PBC (ie, florid duct lesions and granulomas) are not always present. Less specific, but common, features of PBC, which include portal lymphoplasmacytic infiltrates with mild bile duct injury, are features that may be difficult to distinguish from ACR. In such cases, the presence of eosinophils and endotheliitis favors ACR.[21] Because PBC generally recurs months to years after transplantation, the primary differential diagnosis is often LAR or CR (see later discussion). Because bile duct injury is less common in late than early ACR, significant duct injury in the absence of endotheliitis and eosinophils favors recurrent PBC, whereas CPV favors LAR. **Table 1** summarizes histologic features that are helpful in distinguishing ACR from recurrent PBC.

Histopathologic Features of LAR

Histopathologically, there is significant overlap between features of recurrent HCV and ACR. Overall, histologic features favoring recurrent hepatitis C include the monotonous nature of infiltrates with few or rare eosinophils, the absence of duct epithelial and endothelial injury, interface hepatitis with ductular reaction, and presence of lobular inflammation with evidence of hepatocellular injury and death/apoptosis. In contrast, histologic features favoring ACR include mixed infiltrates with eosinophils, prominent bile duct damage, and endotheliitis. Bile duct lymphocytic infiltration might be seen in HCV, but it is generally mild and not accompanied by significant epithelial injury. Similarly, inflammation around the portal veins (perivenulitis) may be present in HCV, but this is generally mild and not associated with morphologic evidence of endothelial cell injury such as lifted endothelium (ie, endotheliitis).[4,22–24]

The distinction between recurrent HCV and LAR is even more difficult, because both are characterized by histologic features of chronic hepatitis. In addition, eosinophils, prominent bile duct damage, and characteristic endotheliitis might not be present in LAR. In such cases, the presence of CPV is a helpful histologic feature. Although CPV may be seen in cases of HCV, it is typically mild and involves only a few hepatic veins. Presence of CPV (with or without necrosis, and with or without central vein endotheliitis) that involves

Table 1
Histologic features of acute rejection versus those of recurrent hepatitis C and PBC

Histologic Feature	Acute Rejection	Recurrent Hepatitis C	PBC
Portal inflammation	Mixed, with activated lymphocytes, plasma cells, neutrophils, and eosinophils. Not nodular	Predominantly lymphocytic, may be nodular. Eosinophils are inconspicuous or few	Lymphoplasmacytic, sparse or dense, may be centered on bile duct
Bile ducts	Variable infiltration by lymphocytes from mild to marked, with epithelial injury from mild to severe	± Mild and focal infiltration by lymphocytes with mild/focal epithelial injury	Variable infiltration by lymphocytes and variable injury from mild to florid duct lesion
Portal vein endotheliitis	Prominent	Absent or mild and focal	Absent
Interface activity	Variable (often seen in moderate to severe acute rejection and in LAR)	Minimal in early recurrence, variable from mild to marked with chronicity	Ductular reaction or interface activity is often present
Lobular activity/injury	May be present in severe acute rejection but also in LAR	Predominant in early recurrence, variable later	Variable. Generally minimal
Apoptotic hepatocytes	Absent to occasional	Frequent	Absent to occasional
CPV (with or without central vein endotheliitis)	May be present in severe acute rejection or LAR	Absent or focal and mild, without endotheliitis	Generally uninvolved

most central veins favors LAR.[15–18,24,25] **Table 1** summarizes histologic features that are helpful in distinguishing ACR from recurrent HCV. The interobserver agreement for the histopathologic diagnosis of ACR versus recurrent HCV is low, even among experienced liver pathologists.[26]

Clinical Consideration in LAR

Careful consideration of clinical factors is important in the differential diagnosis of recurrent HCV versus ACR. The time from transplantation to biopsy, whether there is a history of medication noncompliance or therapeutic dose reduction because of recent illness or infection, liver biochemistry, and HCV RNA levels should be carefully reviewed. If available, the most recent previous biopsy needs to be reviewed in conjunction with the current biopsy.

The distinction between recurrent HCV and ACR is clinically critical because the treatment of one has deleterious effects on the other.[23] Patients with hepatitis C who have been treated for multiple episodes of ACR with high-dose immunosuppressive treatment show an accelerated course of hepatitis C progression with increased risk of allograft cirrhosis and a higher rate of mortality.[27,28] On the other hand, if ACR is left untreated, it may progress to CR.[23] Therefore, in cases of recurrent HCV in which the biopsy features are indeterminate for rejection or a mild ACR cannot be reliably excluded, the uncertainty should be clearly conveyed in the pathology report so that patients are monitored closely and a subsequent biopsy considered if liver enzymes continue to increase.

CR

CR affects only 3% to 5% of liver allografts but is nevertheless still an important cause of late graft dysfunction and failure. Clinically, patients generally present with jaundice and a cholestatic pattern of injury with increase of alkaline phosphatase and γ-glutamyl transferase levels. Most patients with CR have documented episodes of ACR or history of suboptimal immunosuppression. Although advanced CR is considered irreversible and leads to graft loss, early CR is potentially reversible, if diagnosed and treated early.[16,29]

The minimum diagnostic criteria for diagnosis of CR are[29]:

1. Presence of bile duct atrophy/senescence affecting most of the bile ducts, with or without bile duct loss (early CR) or
2. Foam cell obliterative arteriopathy (OA) or
3. Loss of interlobular bile ducts in at least 50% of portal tracts

Bile duct atrophy/senescence is characterized by irregular epithelial spacing, loss of polarity, nuclear atypia, and increased cytoplasmic eosinophilia (**Fig. 3**A). Loss of small arterial branches in the portal tracts has also been reported early in CR. In CR, inflammation is often minimal, and ductular reaction is not typically seen. Similar to other chronic biliary processes, lobular aggregates of pigmented foamy macrophages and canalicular cholestasis are often present (see **Fig. 3**B).[2,30]

Foam Cell OA in CR

Foam cell OA is the pathognomonic feature of CR and is characterized by intimal thickening with accumulation of lipid-laden foamy macrophages, which can cause luminal narrowing and obstruction (see **Fig.** 3C). As the lesion progresses, foamy cells are replaced by proliferating myofibroblasts and fibrosis, which may lead to complete obliteration of lumen and secondary ischemic damage to the parenchyma and bile ducts. Usually, bile duct loss and OA are found together, although cases with only 1 of these features may occur. Because OA primarily affects large and medium-sized arterial branches located in or near the hilum, it is rarely sampled in biopsy specimens. However, the presence of ischemic damage secondary to OA may be appreciated on biopsies. These ischemic changes include centrilobular damage with cholestasis and ballooned and swollen hepatocytes with or without hepatocellular dropout/necrosis. A variable amount of perivenular fibrosis may also develop and is usually mild. In advanced cases, perivenular fibrosis may lead to central vein obliteration and central-to-central or central-to-portal bridging fibrosis.[2,29,30]

Differential Diagnosis in CR

The diagnostic emphasis in biopsy material is particularly placed on presence of bile duct atrophy/senescence or loss. However, bile duct injury or loss can also be seen in drug injury, hepatic artery stricture or thrombosis, and biliary processes such as biliary obstruction, recurrent PBC, and recurrent primary sclerosing cholangitis (PSC). In biliary obstruction, senescent ducts are often seen and therefore should not be used as the only criterion for diagnosing CR in patients with features of obstruction.[16] The presence of ductular reaction and mixed portal inflammation with neutrophils favors obstruction. In contrast, CR has minimal portal inflammation and it is predominantly lymphoplasmacytic. Moreover, although ductular reaction may be seen in recovering cases of CR, it is typically absent in untreated CR. Recurrent PSC is also a stricturing process, which may

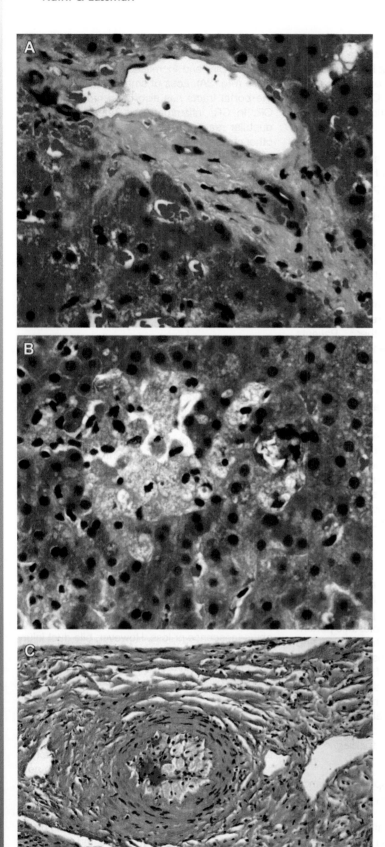

Fig. 3. CR. (*A*) Early CR with senescent duct, characterized by cytoplasmic eosinophilia, unevenly spaced nuclei, nuclear pleomorphism, and only partial lining of bile duct by epithelial cells. There is no ductular reaction or portal infiltrate. (*B*) Cluster of pigmented foamy macrophages within the lobule. (*C*) Foam cell OA characterized by arterial intimal thickening with foamy lipid-laden macrophages. The lumen is nearly completely occluded. This lesion is rarely seen in biopsy material.

result in atrophy/senescence and loss of interlobular bile ducts. However, other features of PSC that are not present in CR include significant portal inflammation, ductular reaction, portal fibrosis, periductal fibrosis, and collagenous scars in place of the bile ducts (Table 2).[31]

Similarly, because both CR and PBC result in bile duct atrophy and ductopenia, distinction on biopsy specimens can be challenging. In general, ductopenia accompanied by portal inflammation favors recurrent PBC over CR. In addition, most cases of PBC are not uniform in appearance, with different portal areas showing various stages of disease. Whereas some portal tracts show absence of bile ducts, others show portal infiltrates and yet others might have florid duct lesions or ductular reaction. This heterogeneity of inflammatory lesions favors recurrent PBC over CR. Furthermore, CR does not generally result in extensive portal bridging fibrosis and, instead, is characterized in its late phases by mild perivenular fibrosis. Therefore, the presence of portal-to-portal bridging fibrosis favors recurrent PBC over CR (see Table 2).

Distinguishing CR from recurrent hepatitis C is generally straightforward. CR is a paucicellular process, with minimal portal fibrosis. This situation is in contrast to chronic hepatitis C, which has portal and lobular lymphoid infiltrates with portal fibrosis (see Table 2). When recurrent HCV and CR coexist, bile duct atrophy and loss may be accompanied by a portal mononuclear cell infiltrate with or without interface and lobular necroinflammatory activity. In such cases, it might be difficult to evaluate for the presence of bile duct damage or loss, and therefore, immunohistochemical (IHC) staining for cytokeratins (eg, cytokeratin 7 or 19) may be helpful in evaluating bile ducts. In the setting of advanced fibrosis from hepatitis C or other causes, the scarring process, neovascularization, and extensive ductular reaction may obliterate the portal areas and obscure the interlobular bile ducts. In such cases, biopsy material may simply be inadequate to evaluate

Table 2
Histologic features of CR versus those of recurrent hepatitis C, PBC, and PSC

Histologic Feature	CR	Recurrent Hepatitis C	PBC	PSC
Portal inflammation	Minimal lymphocytic infiltrate	Nodular lymphocytic aggregates	Variable, from minimal infiltrates similar to CR to inflammatory and destructive lesions	Variable, from minimal infiltrates similar to CR to inflammatory and destructive lesions
Bile ducts	Early CR: atrophy and senescence Late CR: absent	Normal to mild infiltration	May be normal, atrophic, or absent. Inflammatory lesions may be present	May be normal, atrophic, or absent. Periductal fibrosis or collagenous scars may be present
Portal fibrosis	No or minimal fibrous expansion	Variable, portal fibrosis advancing to bridging and cirrhosis	Variable, portal fibrosis advancing to bridging and cirrhosis. May be accompanied by ductular reaction	Variable, portal fibrosis advancing to bridging and cirrhosis. May be accompanied by ductular reaction
Interface activity	None or minimal	Present, variable	Variable	Variable
Ductular reaction	Absent, except in recovering cases	May be present	Generally present	Generally present
Lobular activity/injury	Early CR: none or minimal Late CR: Kupffer cell aggregates, cholestasis, mild perivenular fibrosis	Variable. Apoptotic cells are usually present; small lymphocytic or Kupffer cell aggregates maybe present	May be similar to CR with Kupffer cell aggregates and cholestasis	May be similar to CR with Kupffer cell aggregates and cholestasis

for duct atrophy or loss, and it is our practice to include a diagnostic comment stating that CR cannot be excluded.

In the setting of a recent episode of treated ACR, bile duct damage might persist despite the resolution of portal inflammation and endotheliitis. Therefore, when a biopsy is taken soon after an episode of treated ACR, it might be difficult to ascertain whether presence of bile duct damage represents resolving ACR or evolving CR. Correlation with the clinical finding with special attention to the trend of liver injury tests after treatment may be helpful in this distinction. Because CR is an evolving process, in some cases, several biopsies may be necessary to establish a diagnosis.

PLASMA CELL HEPATITIS

Plasma cell hepatitis (PCH) is a recently described posttransplant histologic pattern of injury. It is characterized by the presence of plasma cell rich portal and lobular inflammatory infiltrates, closely resembling autoimmune hepatitis (AIH) in the native liver (Fig. 4). Many of these cases are associated with centrilobular inflammation with or without necrosis (ie, CPV; see earlier discussion).[32–34]

Many cases of PCH have been reported in patients transplanted for HCV. Some have been reported in the setting of antiviral therapy (pegylated interferon and ribavirin), suggesting that this might be an alloimmune response, which is triggered by interferon-induced stimulation of the host immune system.[35–39] However, this same pattern of injury has been reported in patients with recurrent HCV but no history of antiviral therapy, as well as in patients transplanted for reasons other than HCV.

In a study by Khettry and colleagues,[32] 9 of 92 (10%) patients transplanted for HCV had a plasma cell rich portal, periportal and lobular necroinflammatory activity (ie, PCH) in posttransplant biopsies. Six of these 9 patients (67%) had autoantibodies or increased serum immunoglobulins, suggesting an autoimmune variant of recurrent HCV or a de novo AIH. These patients also had a higher incidence of CPV, with more rapid progression to fibrosis.

However, in another study by Fiel and colleagues,[33] almost all 38 patients with PCH had low titer autoantibodies, and only 14 of 38 patients (37%) had autoantibody titers of 1:40 or greater. Most cases (82%) were associated with suboptimal or recent lowering of immunosuppression, suggesting that PCH represents a form of acute rejection. These patients also had a high incidence of ACR before developing PCH, indicating a propensity for rejection. They had a better outcome when treated with optimization of immunosuppression.

Clearly, PCH is a form of posttransplant immune-mediated injury. Whether it represents LAR, a variant of recurrent HCV, de novo or recurrent AIH might not be significant in terms of clinical management. It seems that regardless of pathophysiology, studies agree that the development of PCH is a negative prognostic factor for graft and patient outcome, and needs to be treated by

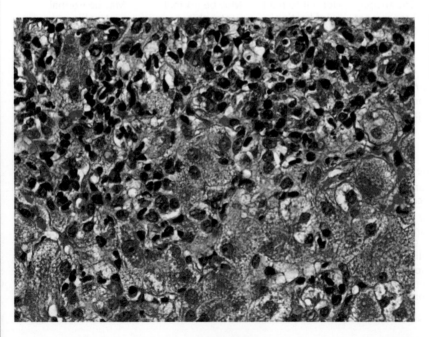

Fig. 4. PCH. Numerous plasma cells are present amongst the portal and periportal inflammatory infiltrate.

immunosuppression.[32–34,40,41] In our practice, we generally report these cases as PCH, with a comment indicating that PCH most likely represents a form of LAR, which, if not treated accordingly, may result in a poor outcome.

IDIOPATHIC POSTTRANSPLANT CHRONIC HEPATITIS

Idiopathic posttransplant chronic hepatitis (IPTH) is a form of posttransplant hepatitis that cannot be attributed to a recognized cause. Patients with IPTH are usually diagnosed on protocol biopsies and are asymptomatic with normal or near normal liver enzymes. The reported incidence is variable, ranging from less than 10% up to approximately 50%.[42–45]

The pathologic features are similar to those of chronic hepatitis in the nontransplant setting. There are mononuclear cell infiltrates in portal tracts, with varying degrees of interface and lobular activity. By definition, bile duct damage and endotheliitis characteristic of rejection are minimal or absent.[45,46]

IPTH should be a diagnosis of exclusion after all other potential causes of hepatitis (infection, drug, autoimmune) and cellular rejection have been ruled out. Newly acquired viral hepatitis B, C, or E should be kept in mind in patients transplanted for reasons other than viral hepatitis. If there is suspicion for hepatitis B infection and the results of serologic studies are not available, an IHC stain for hepatitis B surface antigen may be helpful. Infection with other nonhepatotropic viruses needs to be considered as well. IHC stains for cytomegalovirus (CMV), herpes simplex virus (HSV), adenovirus and in situ hybridization (ISH) for Epstein-Barr virus (EBV) RNA (EBER) may be helpful. A major consideration in cases of IPTH is chronic hepatitis pattern of rejection (ie, LAR). As mentioned earlier, if CPV is present and involves most portal veins, then LAR should be favored.[16,46] In our practice, we do not generally use IPTH as a diagnostic term. Rather, we report these cases as hepatitis, with a comment indicating that this pattern of injury requires clinical correlation to exclude an underlying cause. We recommend a complete serologic workup to exclude viral and AIH (if not already performed). In addition, we recommend correlation with clinical events, such as history of noncompliance, recent reduction in immunosuppression, recent illness interfering with absorption of medication, or new drugs that may either cause drug-induced hepatitis or affect level of immunosuppression.

FIBROSING CHOLESTATIC HEPATITIS

Fibrosing cholestatic hepatitis (FCH) is a rare and aggressive form of viral hepatitis infection, which occurs in patients under severe immunosuppression.[47] It was first described in 1991 by Davies and colleagues[48] in patients transplanted for chronic hepatitis B. Since then, it has been recognized in patients with both hepatitis B and C who are immunocompromised for different reasons, including stem cell and solid organ transplantation and human immunodeficiency virus infection.[48–51] In the liver transplant setting, despite reports of successful treatment in cases of hepatitis B after transplantation,[52] graft loss is still a major concern, particularly with hepatitis C.

Histologic Features of FCH

Histologically, FCH is characterized by marked hepatocellular injury in the form of ballooning change and apoptosis, predominantly in the perivenular zone. Characteristically, there is a paucity of portal and lobular inflammatory infiltrate. Bridging necrosis with parenchymal collapse may be present. There is extensive intracellular and canalicular cholestasis. More advanced cases show marked ductular reaction. Periportal and pericellular/sinusoidal fibrosis is present and may rapidly progress to portal-to-portal bridging fibrosis (Fig. 5).[48,53–57] Box 1 summarizes the clinicopathologic features of FCH.

Differential Diagnosis in FCH

The primary clinical and histologic differential diagnosis of FCH is bile duct obstruction (BDO). Whereas cholestasis and ductular reaction can be seen in both, BDO is not generally accompanied by extensive hepatocellular injury and instead may show prominent portal edema. The diagnosis of FCH is especially difficult when there is concurrent biliary injury, and histology alone may not be sufficient to exclude biliary compromise.[58] Clinically, FCH is usually seen in association with high levels of HCV RNA. It frequently follows immunosuppressive treatment of ACR or is associated with high levels of immunosuppression. Rapidly increasing levels of HCV RNA after a change in the patient's immunosuppressive regimen are a strong clinical indicator of FCH.

Histologically, FCH may also mimic CR with paucity of inflammation in the setting of cholestasis, Kupffer cell aggregates, ballooning hepatocytes, and perivenular fibrosis. In such cases, careful consideration of clinical findings, including presence of high levels of HCV RNA and a history of an increase, rather than a reduction, in

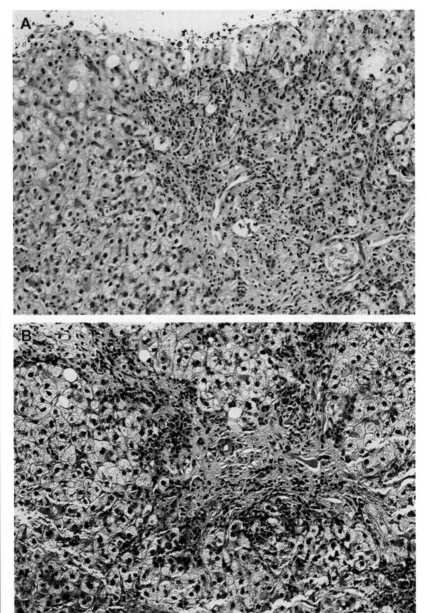

Fig. 5. FCH. (*A*) There is irregular portal expansion and diffuse parenchymal ballooning change. Note the presence of ductular reaction and the relative paucity of inflammatory infiltrate. (*B*) Bridging fibrosis is accompanied by an extensive ductular reaction reminiscent of biliary obstruction.

immunosuppression, helps in establishing a diagnosis of FCH.

In early biopsies when cholestasis is the main feature, drug injury also enters the differential diagnosis. The history of liver injury with recent exposure to a hepatotoxic drug is helpful in making this distinction. Histologic features that favor FCH include extensive hepatocellular injury, rapidly progressive fibrosis despite discontinuation of possible hepatotoxic drug, and documented high viral load. Overall, FCH is best considered a diagnosis of exclusion. Clinical findings must be carefully considered, and imaging studies to rule out BDO should be recommended.

Many reported cases of FCH have been rapidly progressive and fatal. Unlike the usual viral hepatitis, in which the cytopathic injury is mediated by an immune response, FCH is believed to

Box 1
Clinicopathologic features of FCH

Clinical:

- History of recent increase in immunosuppression

Biochemical:

- High viral load (in particular, recent and rapid increase)
- Increased bilirubin levels
- Modest increase of transaminase levels

Histologic:

- Extensively ballooned or swollen hepatocytes
- Prominent cholestasis
- Relative paucity of portal and lobular inflammation
- Ductular reaction
- Periportal and pericellular/sinusoidal fibrosis

result from unchecked viral replication with direct cytolysis of hepatocytes by virus. As described earlier, many cases show a paucity of inflammatory cells.

In a recent study, Moreira and colleagues[59] proposed a novel approach to histologic grading of recurrent HCV in posttransplant setting, which is based on the 4 main histologic features of FCH:

1. Ductular reaction
2. Cholestasis
3. Hepatocyte ballooning
4. Periportal and sinusoidal fibrosis

These investigators report that this system allows accurate identification of FCH and, in addition, enables stratification of patients with recurrent HCV into prognostic categories that are highly predictive of graft loss, independent of necroinflammatory activity and stage.

VIRAL INFECTIONS

Infection is the leading cause of death after OLT. In the following sections, 3 viral pathogens are discussed: CMV, EBV, and hepatitis E. Other potential viruses that may rarely cause infection in liver transplant recipients include HSV, adenovirus, varicella-zoster virus (VZV), and human herpesvirus 6.

CMV INFECTION

CMV is the most common viral pathogen infecting OLT recipients. Without prophylaxis, the overall incidence is 50% to 60%. However, because of the frequent use of antiviral prophylaxis after the transplant, the overall incidence of CMV hepatitis has dramatically decreased, with a reported incidence of 2% to 17%.[60–63] CMV infection nevertheless remains an important consideration in the posttransplant setting when there is graft dysfunction and unexplained increase of liver enzyme levels.

The characteristic histologic appearance of CMV in the allograft liver is the presence of small clusters of neutrophils, known as microabscesses, within the lobules. Small foci of hepatocyte injury, mild lobular disarray, focal lobular necrosis, apoptotic bodies, and Kupffer cell aggregates (microgranulomas) may also be present. The portal tracts are generally only mildly infiltrated by mononuclear or mixed inflammation. The liver biopsy diagnosis depends on the identification of CMV-infected cells, which are usually found near microabscesses. The characteristic CMV inclusions are large eosinophilic, intranuclear inclusions, which are frequently surrounded by a clear halo. Eosinophilic, granular cytoplasmic inclusions may also be present. CMV may infect hepatocytes, endothelial cells, or bile duct epithelial cells (Fig. 6).

Although characteristic CMV inclusions are easy to appreciate, they are not uncommonly absent on routine hematoxylin-eosin sections. Neutrophilic microabscesses are also neither sensitive nor specific, and are not always present.[64] In addition, inflammatory response could be mild or absent because of the patients' immunosuppressive state. We have occasionally encountered allograft biopsies with minimal portal and lobular lymphocytic infiltrates and no inclusions by routine staining in patients with positive serum polymerase chain reaction (PCR) for CMV DNA. Subsequent IHC staining in these patients has shown none to many infected cells with convincing staining for CMV. Therefore, in allograft biopsies with unexplained increase of liver enzyme levels and especially those with the finding of microabscesses, IHC stain for CMV antigen should be considered even in the absence of inclusions or significant inflammation. CMV-infected cells may be sparse, with only 1 or 2 infected cells in a biopsy even by IHC staining.

When CMV is not appreciated by routine stains, diagnostic consideration includes hepatitis caused by hepatotropic viruses such as hepatitis B, C, or E as well as other opportunistic infections. In general, CMV causes less lobular disarray and

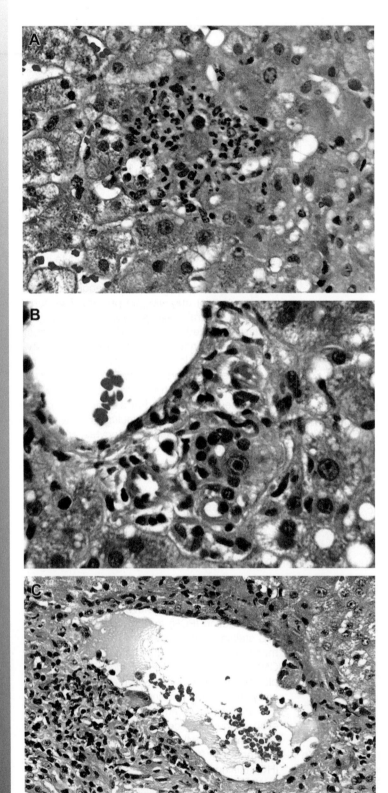

Fig. 6. CMV hepatitis. CMV can infect hepatocytes, endothelial cells, and bile duct epithelial cells. (*A*) A CMV-infected hepatocyte with eosinophilic viral inclusion is seen adjacent to a neutrophilic microabscess. (*B*) A bile duct epithelial cell with a prominent CMV inclusion. (*C*) CMV-infected cells are seen within the endothelium of this portal vein branch.

hepatocyte swelling than hepatitis B virus (HBV) or HCV. In addition, the lobular inflammation seen with HBV and HCV consists primarily of lymphocytes percolating through the sinusoids, whereas in CMV the lobular inflammation often contains neutrophils (ie, microabscesses). Other opportunistic infections such as HSV, VZV, and adenovirus generally cause large areas of coagulative necrosis, whereas CMV causes focal necrosis.

EBV INFECTION

EBV infection is a less frequent cause of allograft dysfunction and is generally secondary to reactivation. More than 90% of adults have had previous exposure to EBV. In liver allografts, EBV infection can cause a broad spectrum of diseases, ranging from mild EBV hepatitis to malignant posttransplant lymphoproliferative disorder (PTLD).

EBV hepatitis usually occurs within the first 6 months after transplantation, with increase of liver enzyme levels. PTLD develops as a consequence of uncontrolled EBV replication secondary to unresolved or recurrent EBV infection. The clinical presentation is generally nonspecific, and the prognosis relies on early diagnosis. Therefore, it is important to be cognizant of EBV hepatitis and PTLD when evaluating allograft liver biopsies.[65]

EBV hepatitis typically shows mild portal and sinusoidal inflammatory infiltrates, consisting predominantly of lymphocytes with occasional admixed plasma cells, eosinophils, and neutrophils. The sinusoidal lymphocytic infiltration has a characteristic linear arrangement or beaded pattern. Most of the lymphocytes are small, but scattered atypical lymphocytes with large irregular nuclei may be present. Histologic features typical of acute hepatitis such as lobular disarray, hepatocyte ballooning, apoptotic bodies, mild steatosis, microgranulomas, and canalicular cholestasis may be present. Foci of interface activity, mild bile duct damage, and subendothelial lymphocytes in portal or central veins can also be seen. PTLD may manifest as a spectrum of histologic findings from early lesions with enlargement of portal tracts by mononuclear infiltrates including atypical lymphocytes to mass lesions that are histologically indistinguishable from lymphoma.[2,66,67]

EBV hepatitis and PTLD must be distinguished from other types of viral hepatitis and from ACR. The presence of mixed portal inflammation, including blastic lymphocytes, smaller lymphocytes, and plasma cells admixed with neutrophils and eosinophils favors ACR. In contrast, portal infiltrates in EBV hepatitis and PTLD are less mixed and include many activated and immunoblastic atypical mononuclear cells. In EBV-related disorders, the portal infiltrates consist predominantly of B cells, whereas in recurrent hepatitis C and rejection, the infiltrates are predominately T cells. In addition, although bile duct damage might be seen in EBV-related disorders, it is mild considering the intensity of portal inflammation. However, in ACR, the greater the degree of portal inflammation, the more severe the bile duct damage.[68,69]

ISH for EBER is a useful test in confirming the diagnosis of an EBV-related disorder. EBER is equally sensitive to PCR in detecting EBV in liver biopsy specimens.[70,71] EBER-positive cells can be sparse, because EBV infects only B lymphocytes, and the infiltrating lymphocytes in EBV are predominantly T lymphocytes. IHC stain for EBV latent membrane protein is less sensitive than ISH for EBER in detecting virus. In approximately 30% of PTLD cases, the presence of EBV cannot be shown. These EBV-negative PTLD cases generally occur later after transplantation and are more likely to be of T-cell origin.[68,72] EBER results need to be interpreted with caution. Occasional EBER-positive cells may be found in the general population as well as in allograft recipients. The significance of this finding is an open question. It is only when EBER-positive cells are present in a biopsy that also shows histopathologic features suggestive of an EBV-related disorder that such a disorder is confirmed. When a liver biopsy shows features suspicious for PTLD, in addition to ISH for EBER, the workup may include IHC stains for B-cell and T-cell markers as well as κ and λ light chains. When these studies are equivocal, molecular and cytogenetic studies including gene rearrangement for immunoglobulins or T-cell receptors may be helpful in establishing a diagnosis of malignancy.

As mentioned earlier for CMV hepatitis, mild EBV hepatitis should also be distinguished from hepatotropic HBV and HCV virus. Features of EBV hepatitis including sinusoidal lymphocytosis and the linear alignment of mononuclear cells in the sinusoids may be seen in other causes of viral hepatitis as well. However, EBV-related disorders are frequently associated with atypical lymphocytes, whereas atypical lymphocytes are unusual in hepatotropic viral hepatitis.

HEPATITIS E INFECTION

Although seropositivity for hepatitis E virus (HEV) has been estimated to be as high as 12% in the United States, HEV is an uncommon cause of clinically apparent acute hepatitis in developed countries. However, progressive and severe chronic hepatitis E infection has recently been identified in immunocompromised patients, including liver transplant patients. The source of infection is often unknown. HEV is potentially treatable with antiviral agents, and therefore awareness of HEV as a cause of chronic hepatitis in transplant patients is important. The histologic features of chronic HEV infection are nonspecific. Therefore, serologic studies for hepatitis E must be considered whenever viral hepatitis is considered.[73–78]

ACUTE ANTIBODY-MEDIATED REJECTION AND ROLE OF C4d

Acute antibody-mediated rejection in the liver is rare and histologically manifests as cholestasis, ductular reaction, thrombosis, neutrophilic infiltration and necrosis.[79] These findings cannot be reliably distinguished from ischemic injury, sepsis and preservation injury. Correlation with the clinical setting such as rapid deterioration of graft function, ABO-incompatibility and presence of donor-specific antibodies is necessary to establish this diagnosis. Immunopositivity for complement component 4d (C4d) has been used for the diagnosis of antibody-mediated rejection in the kidney and other sites, but its role in the liver is not fully established. Diffuse C4d staining of portal vessels including veins, arterioles and capillaries is typically seen in acute antibody-mediated rejection, and diffuse sinusoidal involvement may also be observed.[80] The utility of C4d to distinguish acute cellular rejection and recurrent hepatitis C has also been proposed.[81] However, the specificity and clinical utility of C4d staining remains unclear as it has also been observed in acute cellular rejection, chronic ductopenic rejection, recurrent hepatitis B and C, preservation injury, pediatric autoimmune hepatitis and graft vs. host disease.[82,83] It has been suggested that it can be useful in specific situations such as morphology suspicious for acute antibody-mediated rejection, persistent acute cellular rejection, unresolving ischemia-like changes and presence of donor-specific antibodies.[80] The Banff consensus guidelines for C4d interpretation in liver allografts are expected in 2013.

REFERENCES

1. Banff schema for grading liver allograft rejection: an international consensus document. Hepatology 1997;25:658–63.
2. Wang HL, Anderson CD, Glasgow S, et al. Liver. In: Liapis H, Wang HL, editors. Pathology of solid organ transplantation. Heidelberg (Germany): Springer; 2011. p. 199–314.
3. Batts KP. Acute and chronic hepatic allograft rejection: pathology and classification. Liver Transpl Surg 1999;5:S21–9.
4. Hubscher SG. Transplantation pathology. Semin Liver Dis 2009;29:74–90.
5. Lefkowitch JH. Diagnostic issues in liver transplantation pathology. Clin Liver Dis 2002;6:555–70.
6. Kishi Y, Sugawara Y, Tamura S, et al. Histologic eosinophilia as an aid to diagnose acute cellular rejection after living donor liver transplantation. Clin Transplant 2007;21:214–8.
7. Akamatsu N, Sugawara Y, Tamura S, et al. Late-onset acute rejection after living donor liver transplantation. World J Gastroenterol 2006;12:6674–7.
8. D'Antiga L, Dhawan A, Portmann B, et al. Late cellular rejection in paediatric liver transplantation: aetiology and outcome. Transplantation 2002;73:80–4.
9. Florman S, Schiano T, Kim L, et al. The incidence and significance of late acute cellular rejection (>1000 days) after liver transplantation. Clin Transplant 2004;18:152–5.
10. Junge G, Tullius SG, Klitzing V, et al. The influence of late acute rejection episodes on long-term graft outcome after liver transplantation. Transplant Proc 2005;37:1716–7.
11. Sundaram SS, Melin-Aldana H, Neighbors K, et al. Histologic characteristics of late cellular rejection, significance of centrilobular injury, and long-term outcome in pediatric liver transplant recipients. Liver Transpl 2006;12:58–64.
12. Uemura T, Ikegami T, Sanchez EQ, et al. Late acute rejection after liver transplantation impacts patient survival. Clin Transplant 2008;22:316–23.
13. Hassoun Z, Shah V, Lohse CM, et al. Centrilobular necrosis after orthotopic liver transplantation: association with acute cellular rejection and impact on outcome. Liver Transpl 2004;10:480–7.
14. Krasinskas AM, Demetris AJ, Poterucha JJ, et al. The prevalence and natural history of untreated isolated central perivenulitis in adult allograft livers. Liver Transpl 2008;14:625–32.
15. Demetris AJ. Central venulitis in liver allografts: considerations of differential diagnosis. Hepatology 2001;33:1329–30.
16. Demetris AJ, Adeyi O, Bellamy CO, et al. Liver biopsy interpretation for causes of late liver allograft dysfunction. Hepatology 2006;44:489–501.
17. Hubscher SG. Central perivenulitis: a common and potentially important finding in late posttransplant liver biopsies. Liver Transpl 2008;14:596–600.
18. Adeyi O, Fischer SE, Guindi M. Liver allograft pathology: approach to interpretation of needle biopsies with clinicopathological correlation. J Clin Pathol 2010;63:47–74.
19. Brown RS. Hepatitis C and liver transplantation. Nature 2005;436:973–8.

20. Sylvestre PB, Batts KP, Burgart LJ, et al. Recurrence of primary biliary cirrhosis after liver transplantation: histologic estimate of incidence and natural history. Liver Transpl 2003;9:1086–93.

21. Sebagh M, Farges O, Dubel L, et al. Histological features predictive of recurrence of primary biliary cirrhosis after liver transplantation. Transplantation 1998;65:1328–33.

22. Demetris AJ, Eghtesad B, Marcos A, et al. Recurrent hepatitis C in liver allografts: prospective assessment of diagnostic accuracy, identification of pitfalls, and observations about pathogenesis. Am J Surg Pathol 2004;28:658–69.

23. Burton JR, Rosen HR. Acute rejection in HCV infected liver transplant recipients: the great conundrum. Liver Transpl 2006;12:S38–47.

24. Ziarkiewicz-Wroblewska B, Wroblewski T, Wasiutynski A. Morphological features and differential diagnosis of hepatitis C recurrence after liver transplantation: literature review and results of single transplantation center. Ann Transplant 2008;13: 12–20.

25. Longerich T, Schirmacher P. General aspects and pitfalls in liver transplant pathology. Clin Transplant 2006;20:60–8.

26. Regev A, Molina E, Moura R, et al. Reliability of histopathologic assessment for the differentiation of recurrent hepatitis C from acute rejection after liver transplantation. Liver Transpl 2004;10: 1233–9.

27. McCaughan GW, Zekry A. Impact of immunosuppression on immunopathogenesis of liver damage in hepatitis C virus-infected recipients following liver transplantation. Liver Transpl 2003;9:S21–7.

28. Rosen HR, Shackleton CR, Higa L, et al. Use of OKT3 is associated with early and severe recurrence of hepatitis C after liver transplantation. Am J Gastroenterol 1997;92:1453–7.

29. Demetris A, Adams D, Bellamy C, et al. Update of the International Banff Schema for Liver Allograft Rejection: working recommendations for the histopathologic staging and reporting of chronic rejection. An international panel. Hepatology 2000;31: 792–9.

30. Neil DA, Hubscher SG. Histologic and biochemical changes during the evolution of chronic rejection of liver allografts. Hepatology 2002;35:639–51.

31. Demetris AJ. Distinguishing between recurrent primary sclerosing cholangitis and chronic rejection. Liver Transpl 2006;12:S68–72.

32. Khettry U, Huang WY, Simpson MA, et al. Patterns of recurrent hepatitis C after liver transplantation in a recent cohort of patients. Hum Pathol 2007;38: 443–52.

33. Fiel MI, Agarwal K, Stanca C, et al. Posttransplant plasma cell hepatitis (de novo autoimmune hepatitis) is a variant of rejection and may lead to a negative outcome in patients with hepatitis C virus. Liver Transpl 2008;14:861–71.

34. Demetris AJ, Sebagh M. Plasma cell hepatitis in liver allografts: variant of rejection or autoimmune hepatitis? Liver Transpl 2008;14:750–5.

35. Berardi S, Lodato F, Gramenzi A, et al. High incidence of allograft dysfunction in liver transplanted patients treated with pegylated-interferon alpha-2b and ribavirin for hepatitis C recurrence: possible de novo autoimmune hepatitis? Gut 2007;56: 237–42.

36. Cholongitas E, Samonakis D, Patch D, et al. Induction of autoimmune hepatitis by pegylated interferon in a liver transplant patient with recurrent hepatitis C virus. Transplantation 2006;81:488–90.

37. Kontorinis N, Agarwal K, Elhajj N, et al. Pegylated interferon-induced immune-mediated hepatitis post liver transplantation. Liver Transpl 2006;12: 827–30.

38. Levitsky J, Fiel MI, Norvell JP, et al. Risk for immune-mediated graft dysfunction in liver transplant recipients with recurrent HCV infection treated with pegylated interferon. Gastroenterology 2012;142:1132–9.

39. Merli M, Gentili F, Giusto M, et al. Immune-mediated liver dysfunction after antiviral treatment in liver transplanted patients with hepatitis C: allo or autoimmune de novo hepatitis? Dig Liver Dis 2009;41:345–9.

40. Fiel MI, Schiano TD. Plasma cell hepatitis (de-novo autoimmune hepatitis) developing post liver transplantation. Curr Opin Organ Transplant 2012;17: 287–92.

41. Ward SC, Schiano TD, Thung SN, et al. Plasma cell hepatitis in hepatitis C virus patients post-liver transplantation: case-control study showing poor outcome and predictive features in the liver explant. Liver Transpl 2009;15:1826–33.

42. Sebagh M, Rifai K, Feray C, et al. All liver recipients benefit from the protocol 10-year liver biopsies. Hepatology 2003;37:1293–301.

43. Berenguer M, Rayon JM, Prieto M, et al. Are posttransplantation protocol liver biopsies useful in the long term? Liver Transpl 2001;7:790–6.

44. Burra P, Mioni D, Cecchetto A, et al. Histological features after liver transplantation in alcoholic cirrhotics. J Hepatol 2001;34:716–22.

45. Hübscher SG. What is the long-term outcome of the liver allograft? J Hepatol 2011;55:702–17.

46. Shaikh OS, Demetris AJ. Idiopathic posttransplantation hepatitis? Liver Transpl 2007;13:943–6.

47. Walker N, Apel R, Kerlin P, et al. Hepatitis B virus infection in liver allografts. Am J Surg Pathol 1993;17:666–77.

48. Davies SE, Portmann BC, O'Grady JG, et al. Hepatic histological findings after transplantation for chronic hepatitis B virus infection, including a

unique pattern of fibrosing cholestatic hepatitis. Hepatology 1991;13:150–7.

49. Furuta K, Takahashi T, Aso K, et al. Fibrosing cholestatic hepatitis in a liver transplant recipient with hepatitis C virus infection: a case report. Transplant Proc 2003;35:389–91.

50. Lam PW, Wachs ME, Somberg KA, et al. Fibrosing cholestatic hepatitis in renal transplant recipients. Transplantation 1996;61:378–81.

51. Rosenberg PM, Farrell JJ, Abraczinskas DR, et al. Rapidly progressive fibrosing cholestatic hepatitis-hepatitis C virus in HIV coinfection. Am J Gastroenterol 2002;97:478–83.

52. Jung S, Lee HC, Han JM, et al. Four cases of hepatitis B virus–related fibrosing cholestatic hepatitis treated with lamivudine. J Gastroenterol Hepatol 2002;17:345–50.

53. Wiesner RH, Sorrell M, Villamil F. Report of the first International Liver Transplant Society consensus conference on liver transplantation and hepatitis C. Liver Transpl 2003;9:S1–9.

54. Dixon LR, Crawford JM. Early histologic changes in fibrosing cholestatic hepatitis C. Liver Transpl 2007;13:219–26.

55. Narang TK, Ahrens W, Russo MW. Post-liver transplant cholestatic hepatitis C: a systematic review of clinical and pathological findings and application of consensus criteria. Liver Transpl 2010;16:1228–35.

56. Rubin A, Aguilera V, Berenguer M. Liver transplantation and hepatitis C. Clin Res Hepatol Gastroenterol 2011;35:805–12.

57. Xiao SY, Lu L, Wang HL. Fibrosing cholestatic hepatitis: clinicopathologic spectrum, diagnosis and pathogenesis. Int J Clin Exp Pathol 2008;1:396–402.

58. Satapathy SK, Sclair S, Fiel MI. Clinical characterization of patients developing histologically-proven fibrosing cholestatic hepatitis C post-liver transplantation. Hepatol Res 2011;41:328–39.

59. Moreira RK, Salomao M, Verna EC, et al. The Hepatitis Aggressiveness Score (HAS): a novel classification system for post-liver transplantation recurrent hepatitis C. Am J Surg Pathol 2013;37:104–13.

60. Gane E, Saliba F, Valdecasas GJ, et al. Randomized trial of efficacy and safety of oral ganciclovir in the prevention of cytomegalovirus disease in liver-transplant recipients. The Oral Ganciclovir International Transplantation Study Group [corrected]. Lancet 1997;350:1729–33.

61. Lautenschlager I, Halme L, Hockerstedt K, et al. Cytomegalovirus infection of the liver transplant: virological, histological, immunological, and clinical observations. Transpl Infect Dis 2006;8:21–30.

62. Paya CV, Hermans PE, Wiesner RH, et al. Cytomegalovirus hepatitis in liver transplantation: prospective analysis of 93 consecutive orthotopic liver transplantations. J Infect Dis 1989;160:752–8.

63. Seehofer D, Rayes N, Neumann UP, et al. Changing impact of cytomegalovirus in liver transplantation–a single centre experience of more than 1000 transplantations without ganciclovir prophylaxis. Transpl Int 2005;18:941–8.

64. Lamps LW, Pinson CW, Raiford DS, et al. The significance of microabscesses in liver transplant biopsies: a clinicopathological study. Hepatology 1998;28:1532–7.

65. Langnas AN, Markin RS, Inagaki M, et al. Epstein-Barr virus hepatitis after liver transplantation. Am J Gastroenterol 1994;89:1066–70.

66. Alshak NS, Jiminez AM, Gedebou M, et al. Epstein-Barr virus infection in liver transplantation patients: correlation of histopathology and semiquantitative Epstein-Barr virus–DNA recovery using polymerase chain reaction. Hum Pathol 1993;24:1306–12.

67. Randhawa PS, Markin RS, Starzl TE, et al. Epstein-Barr virus-associated syndromes in immunosuppressed liver transplant recipients. Clinical profile and recognition on routine allograft biopsy. Am J Surg Pathol 1990;14:538–47.

68. Nalesnik MA. Clinical and pathological features of post-transplant lymphoproliferative disorders (PTLD). Springer Semin Immunopathol 1998;20:325–42.

69. Rizkalla KS, Asfar SK, McLean CA, et al. Key features distinguishing post-transplantation lymphoproliferative disorders and acute liver rejection. Mod Pathol 1997;10:708–15.

70. Barkholt L, Reinholt FP, Teramoto N, et al. Polymerase chain reaction and in situ hybridization of Epstein-Barr virus in liver biopsy specimens facilitate the diagnosis of EBV hepatitis after liver transplantation. Transpl Int 1998;11:336–44.

71. Suh N, Liapis H, Misdraji J, et al. Epstein-Barr virus hepatitis: diagnostic value of in situ hybridization, polymerase chain reaction, and immunohistochemistry on liver biopsy from immunocompetent patients. Am J Surg Pathol 2007;31:1403–9.

72. Gottschalk S, Rooney CM, Heslop HE. Post-transplant lymphoproliferative disorders. Annu Rev Med 2005;56:29–44.

73. Haagsma EB, van den Berg AP, Porte RJ, et al. Chronic hepatitis E virus infection in liver transplant recipients. Liver Transpl 2008;14:547–53.

74. Halac U, Béland K, Lapierre P, et al. Chronic hepatitis E infection in children with liver transplantation. Gut 2012;61:597–603.

75. Pischke S, Suneetha PV, Baechlein C, et al. Hepatitis E virus infection as a cause of graft hepatitis in liver transplant recipients. Liver Transpl 2010;16:74–82.

76. Kamar N, Selves J, Mansuy JM, et al. Hepatitis E virus and chronic hepatitis in organ-transplant recipients. N Engl J Med 2008;358:811–7.

77. Kamar N, Garrouste C, Haagsma EB, et al. Factors associated with chronic hepatitis in patients with

hepatitis E virus infection who have received solid organ transplants. Gastroenterology 2011;140: 1481–9.

78. Hoofnagle JH, Nelson KE, Purcell RH. Hepatitis E. N Engl J Med 2012;367:1237–44.

79. Kozlowski T, Rubinas T, Nickeleit V, et al. Liver allograft antibody-mediated rejection with demonstration of sinusoidal C4d staining and circulating donor-specific antibodies. Liver Transpl 2011;17: 357–68.

80. Bellamy CO. Complement C4d immunohistochemistry in the assessment of liver allograft biopsy samples: applications and pitfalls. Liver Transpl 2011; 17:747–50.

81. Schmeding M, Kienlein S, Röcken C, et al. ELISA-based detection of C4d after liver transplantation– a helpful tool for differential diagnosis between acute rejection and HCV-recurrence? TransplImmunol 2010;23:156–60.

82. Ali S, Ormsby A, Shah V, et al. Significance of complement split product C4d in ABO-compatible liver allograft: diagnosing utility in acute antibody mediated rejection. Transpl Immunol 2012;26: 62–9.

83. Bouron-Dal Soglio D, Rougemont AL, Herzog D, et al. An immunohistochemical evaluation of C4d deposition in pediatric inflammatory liver diseases. Hum Pathol 2008;39:1103–10.

Cirrhosis Regression and Subclassification

Pierre Bedossa, MD, PhD[a],*, Guadalupe Garcia-Tsao, MD[b],
Dhanpat Jain, MD[c]

KEYWORDS

• Liver • Cirrhosis • Fibrosis • Regression

ABSTRACT

The end point of liver fibrosis in almost all chronic liver diseases is cirrhosis. Progression to cirrhosis is accompanied by vascular remodeling and regeneration with important functional and hemodynamic consequences that include development of portal hypertension and eventually decompensation and death. Fibrosis can regress following successful treatment of the underlying disease. However, most common fibrosis scoring systems are not equipped for assessing this aspect. Nodule size, septal width and fibrosis area seem to correlate with disease severity and progression in cirrhosis. Classification systems based on nodule size, septal width, and fibrosis area need to be further validated.

OVERVIEW

A common pathologic feature of most chronic liver disease is fibrosis; fibrosis results from an unregulated wound healing response driven by iterative injury shifting the balance of extracellular matrix turnover toward net deposition. This mechanism leads to the progressive replacement of functional hepatic parenchyma by fibrous tissue or extracellular matrix (ECM) that is composed of many different molecules, including highly cross-linked collagen type I/III.[1] The end point of liver fibrosis in almost all chronic liver diseases is cirrhosis, which is characterized by annular fibrosis surrounding hepatocyte nodules.[2] Liver fibrosis and cirrhosis constitute a major global health care burden. Their incidence is increasing with changing patterns of alcohol consumption and increasing rates of obesity and diabetes.[3] It is a major clinical issue because cirrhosis is a risk factor for liver-related complications such as hepatocellular carcinoma (HCC) and death.[4]

The switch from a lobular to a nodular organization is only one part of the morphologic spectrum observed in cirrhosis because angiogenesis, vascular remodeling, sinusoidal capillarization, perisinusoidal fibrosis, and loss of metabolic zonation also develop in this setting with important functional consequences on liver physiology, such as portal hypertension and liver decompensation. Because of this complete morphologic disorganization and the associated major biochemical changes, the dogma prevailing in the literature until recently was that fibrosis, and even cirrhosis, was irreversible and the best hope therapeutically would be to halt progression. Subsequent mounting evidence both in animal models and in humans has provided further support that liver fibrosis and even cirrhosis can regress or even completely revert to normal architecture, either on cessation of the cause of liver injury or treatment of the underlying disease.[5,6]

EVIDENCE FOR CIRRHOSIS REGRESSION

Although it is now well accepted that early to moderate fibrosis can regress and possibly even resolve in several liver diseases, the concept of cirrhosis regression is more challenging.[6] The landmark paper by Perez-Tamayo[7] in 1979 first described evidence in both animal models and human disease for reversal of fibrosis and cirrhosis. In experimental models such as fibrosis induced by chronic carbon tetrachloride (CCl4) intoxication or bile duct ligation in rat, the arrest of fibrogenic stimulus induces reversion of liver fibrosis with

[a] Department of Pathology, Beaujon Hospital and Clichy, University Denis Diderot, Clichy, Paris 7, France;
[b] Section of Digestive Diseases, Department of Medicine, Yale University School of Medicine, New Haven, CT, USA; [c] Department of Pathology, Yale University School of Medicine, New Haven, CT 06520-8023, USA
* Corresponding author.
E-mail address: pierre.bedossa@bjn.aphp.fr

Surgical Pathology 6 (2013) 295–309
http://dx.doi.org/10.1016/j.path.2013.03.006
1875-9181/13/$ – see front matter © 2013 Elsevier Inc. All rights reserved.

surgpath.theclinics.com

virtually normal liver histology as an end point. Later, Wanless and colleagues[8] presented serial biopsies from a patient with hepatitis B following antiviral treatment that showed apparent regression of hepatitis B with a shift from fully developed cirrhosis to incomplete septal cirrhosis. In this landmark paper, Wanless and colleagues[8] also reported livers removed at transplantation having cirrhosis or incomplete septal cirrhosis with complete description of histologic parameters that suggest progression or regression of fibrosis. Thereafter, isolated reports have been published with biopsy-proven regression of cirrhosis of various origins, including hepatitis C, hepatitis B, and autoimmune cirrhosis, following disease-specific therapy.[9] The most fascinating demonstration of the reversibility of cirrhosis comes from studies analyzing large cohorts of patients with hepatitis C virus (HCV) or hepatitis B virus (HBV) cirrhosis effectively treated with antiviral regimens.[10–13] In several of these studies, patients have been followed with serial liver biopsies performed with a sufficient time interval. The largest of these studies was reported by Poynard and colleagues,[14] who retrospectively pooled individual data from several randomized chronic hepatitis C treatment trials, including more than 3000 patients with pretreatment and posttreatment liver biopsies in a mean time of 2 years. Reversal of cirrhosis was observed in 49% of patients with baseline diagnosis of cirrhosis. Other studies assessing regression of cirrhosis after sustained viral response (SVR) following antiviral therapy and longer time interval between paired biopsies showed even higher cirrhosis regression rates (60% after a mean 6 years after SVR). This finding suggests that the longer the follow-up, the higher the percentage of cirrhosis regression.[13] However, treated patients with SVR are still at risk of HCC development, although the risk becomes lower. In the study of George and colleagues,[12] 2 patients with cirrhosis developed HCC during follow-up despite regression of cirrhosis following treatment.

In patients achieving long-term HBV replication suppression with nucleos(t)ide analogues, regression of cirrhosis has been shown in more than 60% of patients subjected to a protocol liver biopsy following 3 to 6 years of treatment.[15,16] Regression of cirrhosis with other causes is also plausible but less well investigated, frequently being based on small, retrospective studies or case reports. Conversion of micronodular to macronodular cirrhosis was reported in 1983 by Fauerholdt and colleagues[17] in a controlled trial of prednisolone in patients with alcoholic cirrhosis. Also, there are several reports of cirrhosis regression in autoimmune hepatitis after treatment with prednisolone

and azathioprine,[18,19] hereditary hemochromatosis following venesection,[20] secondary biliary cirrhosis after biliary drainage of choledocal obstruction, and occasional cases of Wilson disease, all proved by liver biopsy.[21] A common theme to these observations is that cirrhosis regression occurs only following successful treatment of the underlying disease, making elimination of the aggressor the best antifibrotic treatment. Nonalcoholic fatty liver disease (NAFLD) is, to date, the exception to this rule. None of the therapies that ameliorated insulin resistance, hepatic oxidative stress, and steatosis, including bariatric surgery, had a clear effect on fibrosis.[22]

In addition to treating the cause of chronic liver disease, the introduction of pharmacologic agents capable of reducing scarring would represent a major therapeutic advantage. Although there have been significant advances in understanding of the pathogenesis of liver fibrosis enabling identification of potential therapeutic targets, there are still major issues limiting clinical application of antifibrotic therapies.[23]

EVALUATION OF FIBROSIS IN REGRESSING CIRRHOSIS

One major issue pertaining to the regression of cirrhosis is the reliability of methods to measure changes in fibrosis longitudinally. Although assessment of liver fibrosis with liver biopsy remains the current reference standard for quantifying fibrosis, it is, as such, an imperfect gold standard. Sampling error can produce significant variation in results and the size of the biopsy specimen has also been shown to be an important factor in this issue.[24,25] However, liver biopsy in cirrhotic patients is usually small because of fragmentation and the use of a transjugular route. Another issue regarding evaluation of regression of cirrhosis pertains to most common fibrosis scoring systems, such as the Ishak, Batts and Ludwig, or METAVIR staging systems, being developed before the idea of fibrosis regression gained importance and not being equipped for assessing this aspect, in which peculiar histologic features may be observed (discussed later).[26,27]

Based on the current limitations of liver biopsy, a key requirement for future diagnostics of cirrhosis regression assessment is the development of reliable and accurate noninvasive biomarkers of liver fibrosis. Alternatives to the liver biopsy have been developed, including transient elastography and serum marker panels. Although these approaches have progressively gained acceptance as an adjunct for diagnosing cirrhosis, these have not been fully validated for assessing the dynamics of liver fibrosis, especially longitudinal evaluation of fibrosis regression.[28]

Clinical outcomes may be more reliable as a proof of regression of disease. Although the clinical meaningfulness of cirrhosis regression in patients with HBV receiving effective antiviral treatment is still unknown, the long-term clinical response to interferon treatment in patients with liver fibrosis related to chronic viral B infection has recently been addressed in a large meta-analysis. Interferon treatment decreased the risk of clinical hepatic-related events and cirrhotic complications with the greatest benefit seen in patients with sustained response.[29] In patients with HCV there is evidence that regression of cirrhosis has significant clinical benefits, and studies also support the association between SVR and improved clinical outcomes. Mallet and colleagues[30] described a cohort of 96 patients with HCV cirrhosis who underwent repeat liver biopsy following interferon-based treatment. The subgroup that attained SVR had significantly fewer liver-related deaths and events compared with nonresponders. Moreover, no patients reported to have regression of cirrhosis on repeated biopsies reported liver-related deaths or events.

PATHOPHYSIOLOGIC MECHANISMS SUSTAINING CIRRHOSIS REGRESSION

From a mechanistic perspective, several biologic processes have to participate in cirrhosis regression, the evidence of which is mainly derived from experimental models.

Morphometric analysis of paired biopsies in cases with cirrhosis regression has shown a significant decrease of fibrous tissue amount.[13] This decrease is mainly caused by ECM enzymatic digestion. However, ECM molecules are highly stabilized and cross-linked molecules that are insensitive to most human proteases except matrix metalloproteinases (MMPs), which efficiently cleave collagens and other components of the extracellular matrix. This enzyme family is composed of different calcium-dependent and zinc-dependent enzymes, each being specific for a group of ECM components, interstitial collagenases (MMP-1, MMP-8), gelatinases (MMP-2, MMP-9), stromelysins (MMP-3, MMP-7, MMP-10, MMP-11), membrane type (MMP-14, MMP-15, MMP-16, MMP-17, MMP-24, MMP-25), and metalloelastases (MMP-12).[31] Increased collagenase activity is a primary pathway of fibrosis resolution. Withdrawal of the causal source of the chronic injury (eg, HBV, HCV) results in decreased ECM production and increased collagenase activity responsible for matrix degradation.[32] The cellular origin of MMP production during liver fibrosis has been assigned mainly to hepatic stellate cells and activated macrophages/Kupffer cells but their relative contribution remains unknown.[33,34] MMP activation is balanced by an inactivation mechanism, namely the binding, in a specific ratio, to a group of inhibitors known as tissue inhibitors of metalloproteinases (TIMPs). During fibrosis regression, increased activity of collagen-degrading enzymes correlates with decreased TIMPs.[35] Therefore, a sophisticated mechanism regulates the shift between synthesis and degradation of ECM with, on one side, posttranslational activation of MMPs through proteolytic cleavage under the control of the microenvironment, and, on the other side, their inactivation through binding with TIMPs.[36] Subsequent mechanistic studies aiming to alter the TIMP/MMP balance have confirmed the powerful influence this ratio has on the development and resolution of fibrosis.

Once ECM has been degraded, activated hepatic stellate cells (HSCs) progressively disappear. HSCs are considered to play a major role in the development of liver fibrosis. HSCs are perisinusoidal cells that normally reside in the space of Disse and contain numerous retinoid and lipid droplets.[37] In response to injury, quiescent HSCs downregulate retinoid storage, acquire contractility, and get transformed into collagen type I+ α-SMA+ (Smooth muscle action) myofibroblasts.[38] Resolution of stellate cell activation represents an essential step toward reversibility of fibrosis. Whether these activated HSCs reverse to a quiescent phenotype or die by apoptosis or senescence during fibrosis regression is a matter of debate.[39–41] With regards to this hypothesis, HSCs, in their myofibroblastic phenotype, express different cell death receptors, such as CD95 and TNF-related apoptosis related ligand (TRAIL) receptor.[39,42] Stellate cell apoptosis has been documented during recovery after experimental liver injury such as bile duct ligation or CCl4 intoxication.[35]

There is strong evidence that liver cell regeneration is also a crucial condition needed for cirrhosis to regress. Morphologic studies suggest that the succession from micronodular to macronodular cirrhosis represents the early anatomic step in cirrhosis regression in humans.[8,17] The mechanism that supports this transformation is hepatocyte regeneration. This transition is also observed in animal models of cirrhosis regression with incomplete septal cirrhosis as an advanced stage of cirrhosis regression.[43] In this scheme, it is postulated that regeneration of liver cells acts through distension and rupture of fibrous septa leading to a partial recovery of the lobular architecture. The functional demonstration of liver cell regeneration as a driver of cirrhosis regression has been shown in an animal model of liver cirrhosis in which hepatocyte regeneration has been forced through telomerase gene delivery in liver cells.[44] However, liver regeneration is not a universal mechanism in cirrhosis. Hepatocyte regeneration needs the internal potential of liver cells to divide and the cessation of necroinflammatory processes.[45] Necroinflammation, through production of various cytokines and growth factors, acts as a brake for liver regeneration. Thus, an efficient treatment of disorders such as antiviral drug therapy for viral hepatitis, allows the arrest of necroinflammation and liver regeneration to occur, a mechanism that may favor cirrhosis regression.

Whether cirrhosis and the accompanying vascular remodeling may reach a point at which the lesion is irreversible has been debated. The areas of fibrosis that do not undergo remodeling are extensively cross-linked and rich in elastin fibers, suggesting that ECM cross-linking might represent a 'point of no return' in cirrhosis. Reversibility of fibrosis depends on the age of the accumulated fibrillar ECM. Cirrhosis that has been recently constituted, as characterized by the presence of thin and edematous fibers, often in the presence of a diffuse inflammatory infiltrate, seems to be fully reversible, whereas, in long-standing cirrhosis, thick highly cross-linked collagen fibrils and elastic fibers may prevent its degradation.[6] Regarding the potential for cirrhosis to reverse, there is a rationale to categorize cirrhosis in different histologic subgroups (discussed later).

HISTOPATHOLOGIC PATTERN OF REGRESSING CIRRHOSIS

There are few studies focusing on the histopathologic pattern of regressing fibrosis.[8] Such studies should ideally be based on sequential biopsies to assess morphologic patterns in their dynamic context.[9,13,46] As mentioned previously, cirrhosis regression is associated with a net decrease in the amount of fibrous tissue that can easily be shown by morphometric measurement of fibrosis area (Fig. 1). One of the representative features is a major thinning of fibrous septa that may be reduced to a cluster of very thin collagen fibers (Fig. 2). Together with septal thinning, there is disappearance of shunting neovessels that develop as a result of angiogenesis associated with fibrogenesis. Thin septa of regressing cirrhosis usually lack vessels or contain only a few residual capillaries that may not function as shunting vessels (Fig. 3). Thereafter, septa become incomplete (incomplete septal cirrhosis) or may disappear. Regression of fibrosis is associated with a partial or full restoration of the lobular organization. Portal tracts and central veins are present, some of them containing an incomplete portal triad (Fig. 4). Portal vein thrombosis may halt this reshaping of

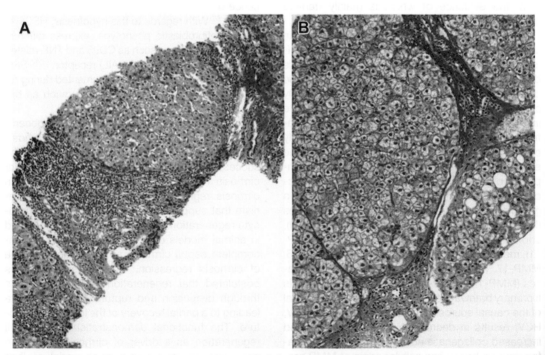

Fig. 1. (A) Hepatitis C cirrhosis before treatment. Well-formed regenerative nodules with annular and broad fibrous septa containing chronic inflammatory infiltrate. (B) Biopsy of the same patient, 3 years after antiviral therapy and SVR showing features of regressing cirrhosis. Nodular organization is still visible but portal tracts are connected by thinner fibrous septa.

Fig. 2. Regressing cirrhosis showing portal tracts interconnected by thin fibrous septa (picro sirius red stain).

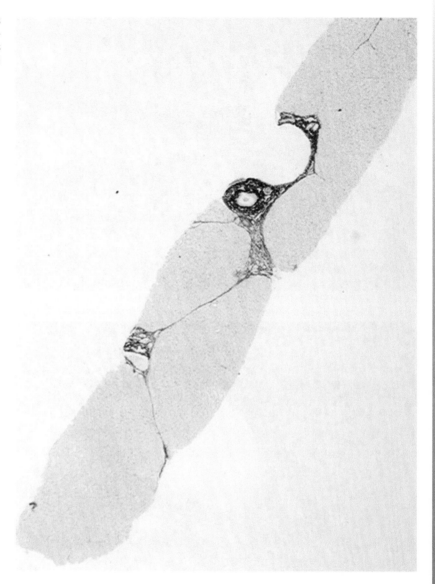

lobular organization. Nodular organization may persist despite the disappearance of fibrous septa leading to a pattern that closely resembles nodular regenerative hyperplasia. Whether perisinusoidal fibrosis and sinusoidal capillarization regress with reversion of the endothelial capillary to a normal sinusoidal phenotype is not clear. Recent studies suggest that this pattern may regress more inconsistently.[13] By contrast, ductular proliferation, a feature associated with fibrosis progression, quickly disappears in regressing cirrhosis. In addition, although metabolic zonation is generally lost in cirrhosis, reversion is associated with restitution of normal lobular enzymatic zonation. The histologic features of cirrhosis regression are listed in **Box 1**.

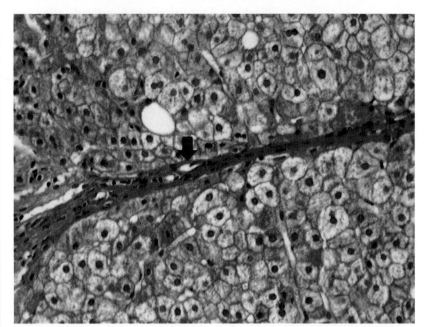

Fig. 3. Higher magnification of regressing fibrous septa. Septum is reduced to a few collagen bundles with residual capillaries (*arrow*).

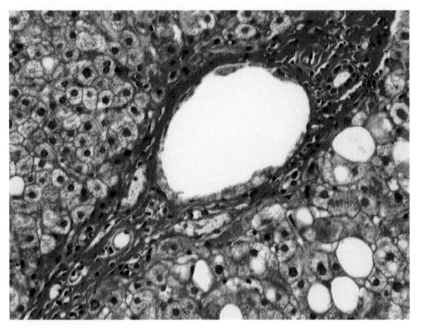

Fig. 4. Restored portal tract after cirrhosis regression (hepatitis C, 5 years after SVR). Portal tract is elongated by fibrous extensions, but bile duct, artery, and vein are noticeable.

Box 1
Histologic features of regressed cirrhosis
Thin or incomplete fibrous septa
No shunting vessels expanding from portal tract
Partial or full restoration of lobular architecture
Some portal tract or central vein visible
Lack of ductular proliferation
Restoration of enzymatic lobular zonation (eg, CYP-2-E1, glutamine synthase)

Need for Subclassification of Cirrhosis

Disease progression in liver leads to increased hepatocytic injury and increasing fibrosis, and hence all staging systems for chronic liver diseases of different causes use progressive fibrosis as the key feature. In all these staging systems, cirrhosis constitutes the most advanced stage because it often leads to portal hypertension, progressive liver cell failure, decompensation, and death. Cirrhosis had been considered irreversible and was often referred to as end-stage liver disease; however, as discussed earlier, it has become increasingly evident that liver fibrosis and remodeling is a dynamic process and even cirrhosis can regress. A group of prominent liver pathologists recently suggested that the concept of cirrhosis has become outdated and should be abandoned.[47] However, it could be argued that cirrhosis represents a significant landmark in the stage of various chronic liver disorders with important clinicopathologic connotations.[47] Although a change in the approach to advanced liver disease is necessary, it may be easier to recognize various subgroups within cirrhosis rather than completely change the terminology. Because the response to treatment in patients with cirrhosis caused by viral hepatitis B or C varies markedly, with some showing remarkable improvement of advanced fibrosis, some remaining stable, and others continuing to deteriorate, it is necessary to stage the degree of fibrosis within a cirrhotic liver. This need will become even more obvious with the advent of antifibrotic agents.

Although the clinical staging of cirrhosis based on factors that predict death has acquired more granularity and has allowed the identification of those with the greatest need for liver transplantation, a histologic staging of cirrhosis has lagged behind.

Clinical Subclassification of Cirrhosis

Cirrhosis has been classified clinically into compensated and decompensated cirrhosis.[48] Decompensation is defined by the clinically detected onset of ascites, variceal hemorrhage, hepatic encephalopathy, or jaundice, all of these complications resulting from portal hypertension and/or liver insufficiency. The median survival for patients with decompensated cirrhosis is estimated to be about 2 years, compared with more than 12 years in those with compensated cirrhosis.[49] Other clinical staging systems for patients with cirrhosis, like the Child-Pugh scoring system and the Model for End-stage Liver Disease (MELD) have also been in extensive clinical use for many years.[48]

Among various clinical parameters, portal hypertension is the earliest and most important consequence of cirrhosis and leads to most of the complications of cirrhosis that define decompensation.[50,51] The hepatic venous pressure gradient (HVPG), a measure of portal hypertension, has now been well established as an indicator of clinical severity of chronic liver disease and cirrhosis. Normal HVPG is 3 to 5 mm Hg and an HVPG of 6 mm Hg or greater defines portal hypertension. In patients with chronic liver disease (METAVIR stages 0–3), specifically posttransplant

hepatitis C, an HVPG of 6 mm Hg or greater has been shown to predict the development of complications of cirrhosis better than histologic fibrosis staging.[52] In patients with cirrhosis, an HVPG of 10 mm Hg or greater has been shown to be the best predictor of the development of complications of portal hypertension (varices, variceal hemorrhage, ascites, and encephalopathy),[49] and hence this threshold of 10 mm Hg is also referred to as clinically significant portal hypertension (CSPH). Studies show that HVPG is generally 12 mm Hg or greater in patients with variceal hemorrhage and ascites.[50,51] However, variceal hemorrhage does not occur when the HVPG is reduced to less than 12 mm Hg.[53] In patients with variceal hemorrhage, an HVPG greater than 20 mm of Hg is a predictor of poor prognosis.[49,54]

Thus clinical staging systems can be based on HVPG measurements, as proposed by Garcia-Tsao and colleagues.[48] However, HVPG measurements are obtained through an invasive procedure and reliable measurements require adherence to standards that are currently only followed in a small number of centers. One of the advantages of HVPG measurements is that, in the same procedure, liver specimens can be obtained via transjugular biopsy. This technique has allowed the performance of histologic-hemodynamic correlations in cirrhosis; however, in most centers where HVPG is not routinely performed, subclassification of cirrhosis loses granularity, particularly in the compensated patient.

Rationale for Pathologic Subclassification of Cirrhosis

Although liver biopsy is an invasive procedure, it remains the gold standard for staging chronic liver disease and for establishing the diagnosis of a variety of liver disorders. Several noninvasive methods of assessing fibrosis stage are increasingly being used and could replace liver biopsy in some settings.[55–58] However, liver biopsy has the advantage of providing more information regarding the pathophysiology of a disorder and it can be reviewed retrospectively for any histologic features deemed to be important. Liver biopsies are frequently used to monitor response to therapy in patients with chronic liver disease, both clinically and in clinical trials. Many of the current trials are performed in patients with cirrhosis, and the identification of histologic features that indicate cirrhosis progression or improvement would be extremely useful; the need for a histologic subclassification of cirrhosis cannot be overstated.

As mentioned earlier, in patients with compensated cirrhosis, the degree of CSPH predicts the development of clinical decompensation. Because a distortion of liver architecture is mainly responsible for the increased portal pressure in cirrhosis, it might be assumed that histologic characteristics could also predict the degree of portal hypertension and, thus, predict the development of outcomes.

Different groups of investigators have tried to analyze structural changes in liver histology that correlate with portal pressure and hence correlate with the severity of chronic liver disease, including cirrhosis. Histologic features that have been evaluated include the presence of central venules, size of cirrhotic nodules, width of fibrous septa separating the cirrhotic nodules, area of fibrosis, loss of portal tracts, sinusoidal and pericentral fibrosis, necroinflammatory activity, steatosis, and capillarization of sinusoids. Of these, nodule size, septal width, and/or fibrosis area seem to correlate with disease severity and progression in cirrhosis.[59-64] This makes sense pathophysiologically as well. With increasing severity of liver disease, the amount of fibrosis increases and parenchymal mass of hepatocytes decreases. If this were to occur uniformly across the liver, early disease would be characterized by large nodules, thin septa, and a smaller fibrosis area (Fig. 5). With advanced cirrhosis, the cirrhotic nodules are expected to become smaller, septa to become wider, and fibrosis area to increase (see Fig. 5). Along similar lines, a reported case of conversion from micronodular to macronodular cirrhosis was associated with clinical improvement.[17]

This response was recognized initially by a group of prominent liver pathologists (the Laennec group) when they proposed a classification of cirrhosis based on the presence of small nodules and septal thickness. This classification has been called the Laennec system (Table 1) for the staging of cirrhosis into 3 subcategories of the META-VIR cirrhotic stage (stage 4), as follows[65]:

Subcategory 1: (4a) mild cirrhosis; definite or probable cirrhosis, 1 broad septum allowed
Subcategory 2: (4b) moderate cirrhosis; at least 2 broad septa, but no very broad septa, and less than half of the biopsy with small nodules
Subcategory 3: (4c) severe cirrhosis; at least 1 very broad septum, or more than half of the biopsy with minute nodules

Septa were defined as broad when the thickness was equivalent to the size of the nodules, and as very broad when the thickness was greater than the size of the nodules. At first, Wanless and

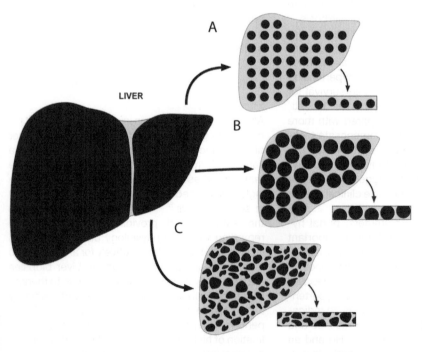

Fig. 5. Rationale for the impact of nodule size, septal width, and area of fibrosis on the severity of cirrhosis. With increasing severity of the liver disease, the amount of fibrosis increases and parenchymal mass of hepatocytes decreases. If this were to occur in a uniform way in the liver, advanced disease would be represented by smaller cirrhotic nodules, wider septa, and more fibrosis (A), whereas milder disease would be represented by larger nodules, thin septa, and less fibrosis area (B). The corresponding biopsies would appear as shown on the side. In reality, this occurs in a nonuniform way and the biopsies show variations in nodule size, nodule contours, and septal width (C), and the biopsies may appear as shown on the side.

Table 1
Laennec system compared with the proposed Jain-Garcia system of cirrhosis subclassification

	Laennec System	Jain-Garcia System
Mild cirrhosis (4a)	Definite or probable cirrhosis, thin septa, 1 broad septum allowed	1. Thin septa with large or mixed nodules 2. Intermediate septa with large nodules
Moderate cirrhosis (4b)	At least 2 broad septa, but no very broad septum	1. Intermediate septa with mixed nodules 2. Thin septa with small nodules
Severe cirrhosis (4c)	At least 1 very broad septum, or many minute nodules	1. Thick septa with any size nodules 2. Intermediate septa with small nodules

Laennec system: this can be established only on biopsies of adequate size. The septal thickness is defined as broad when the size is equivalent to the size of the nodules, and very broad when it is greater than the size of the nodules.

Jain-Garcia system: thin septa, less than 0.1 mm; intermediate septa, 0.1 to 0.2 mm; thick septa, greater than 0.2 mm; small nodules, less than 1 mm; large nodules, greater than 2 mm.

The type of predominant (greater than two-thirds) septa or nodules in the biopsy is taken into account to classify the biopsy, which is otherwise considered mixed. Intermediate and mixed septa are considered the same.

colleagues[65] applied this system in a study assessing fibrosis in patients with hemochromatosis undergoing treatment.[66] A recent study from Korea validated these findings in a cohort of patients with mostly alcoholic cirrhosis in which they showed excellent correlation of the Laennec system with not only HVPG but also with a cirrhosis staging system proposed by D'Amico and colleagues,[67] as well as with the severity of varices and ascites.[68]

This concept had a good pathophysiologic basis and many subsequent studies have used various modifications of the system. One study that systematically analyzed the liver biopsies of 43 patients with compensated cirrhosis mostly caused by chronic hepatitis C showed that, among various histologic parameters, only nodule size and septal width correlated with HVPG.[64]

- The study showed that patients with small nodules and thick septa were more likely to have CSPH defined as an HVPG greater than 10 mm Hg.
- All 22 patients with thick septa and 12 of 13 patients with small nodules had CSPH, and all 8 patients with both small nodules and thick septa had HVPG of 20 mm Hg or greater.
- CSPH was absent in all patients with thin septa but lacking small nodules (n = 4).

Although the study was based on subjective assessment of nodule size and septal width (Fig. 6), it was estimated that small nodules were less than 1 mm, large nodules were greater than 2 mm, thin septa were less than 0.2 mm, and thick septa were greater than 0.4 mm.

A subsequent study by Kumar and colleagues[61] with a similar number of cases but representing patients with cirrhosis mostly caused by hepatitis B validated these findings. In this study, all patients with small nodules (n = 15) or thick septa (n = 18) had CSPH.

Based on their findings, Kumar and colleagues[61] designed a scoring system and subdivided the patients into mild and severe cirrhosis based on these two parameters. This classification based on nodule size and septal width is similar to Laennec system; however, the histologic criteria have been better defined and a modified version is shown in Table 1 along with clinical correlations in Table 2.

Another histologic feature that has been correlated with portal pressure in cirrhosis is the loss of portal tracts,[63] although this has not been confirmed in other studies[61,62] and this histologic feature has been deemed to be difficult to assess.[59] Although loss of portal tracts and central veins have a theoretic physiologic basis in predicting the severity of cirrhosis, these are histologic features that are complicated to assess and therefore it is difficult to incorporate them into any staging/scoring system. Increased capillarization of sinusoids has also been shown to correlate with the development of portal hypertension and liver dysfunction in chronic liver disease; however, this feature is also difficult to quantify in practice.[69]

The extent of liver fibrosis is probably the most important histologic feature that directly correlates with advancing liver disease and it indicates increased resistance to blood flow, structural alterations of liver architecture, and vascular shunts. Studies show that increasing fibrosis correlates significantly with increasing HVPG through all stages of chronic liver diseases, in the absence of cirrhosis,[53] in patients with compensated cirrhosis,[61] and even in those with CSPH.[65]

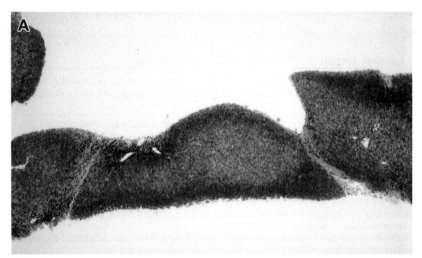

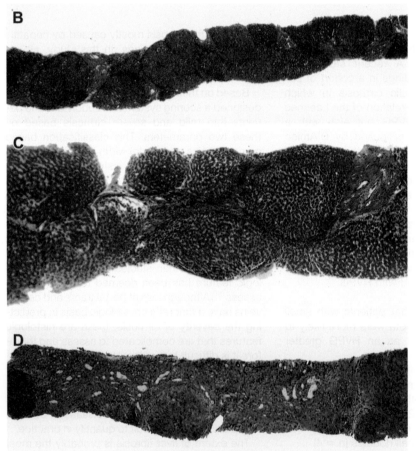

Fig. 6. Representative liver biopsies showing varying sizes of nodules and septa (trichrome stain). (A) Mild cirrhosis (stage 4a) with large nodules with thin septa. (B) Moderate cirrhosis (stage 4b) with mixed nodules with intermediate septa. (C) Moderate cirrhosis (stage 4b) with a liver biopsy showing small nodules with thin septa. (D) Severe cirrhosis (stage 4c) with small nodules with thick septa.

Calvaruso and colleagues[59] showed that the area of fibrosis expressed as the area occupied by collagen as a proportion of total biopsy area referred to as collagen proportionate area (CPA) independently correlated with HVPG and was better than the Ishak fibrosis score.

The study included 115 patients with post-transplant recurrent hepatitis C with varying degrees of

Table 2
Proposed subclassification of cirrhosis (Jain-Garcia system)

	4a	4b	4c
Clinical	Compensated Cirrhosis		Decompensated Cirrhosis
	No varices	Varices	Variceal hemorrhage, encephalopathy, ascites
HVPG (mm Hg)	6–10	10–12	>12
1. Histology	1. Thin septa with large or mixed nodules 2. Intermediate septa with large nodules	1. Intermediate septa with mixed nodules 2. Thin septa with small nodules	1. Thick septa with nodules of any size 2. Intermediate septa with small nodules
2. Histologic score	<4	4	>4
Fibrosis (%)	<10	10–30	>30

Score: Septae	Score: Nodules
Thin septae (<0.1 mm) = 1 Intermediate septae (0.1–0.2 mm) = 2 Thick septae (>0.2 mm) = 4	Large nodules (>2 mm) = 1 Mixed nodules = 2 Small nodules (<1 mm) = 3

The type of predominant (greater than two-thirds) septa or nodules in the biopsy is taken into account to classify the biopsy, which is otherwise considered mixed. Intermediate and mixed septa are considered the same.

fibrosis (Ishak stage 0–6), including 23 patients with cirrhosis or early/precirrhosis.

The CPA showed good correlation with HVPG:

- The median CPA in patients with Ishak score of 6 (cirrhosis) was 17% (range 13%–45%).
- The median CPA for patients with HVPG less than 6 mm Hg was 4.1% and, for patients with 6 mm Hg or greater, was 13.8% (P<.0001).
- The best cutoff value of CPA for portal hypertension (≥6 mm Hg) was 7.2% with a sensitivity of 80% and specificity of 79%.
- The CPA for patients without and with CSPH was 6% and 17.3% respectively (P<.0001).
- The best cutoff value of CPA for CSPH (≥10 mm Hg) was 12.5% with a sensitivity of 78% and specificity of 86%.

This study showed that the extent of fibrosis correlates independently with HVPG, even in the subgroup of patients with cirrhosis.

Another study that specifically analyzed only biopsies of cirrhotic livers (n = 42) for various histologic features and extent of fibrosis by digital image analysis also confirmed that fibrosis area independently correlated with HVPG.

- The median fibrosis area in the study by Sethasine and colleagues[60] in patients with CSPH was 12.6% compared with 27% in those without CSPH.

- Except for 1 patient, all those with a fibrosis area less than 15% had an HVPG less than 10 mm Hg.
- Even within the group of patients with CSPH (≥10 mm Hg) there was correlation between increasing fibrosis and HVPG.

Thus, fibrosis estimated quantitatively by digital analysis remains one of the strongest predictors of HVPG and severity of cirrhosis.

In the same study based on quantitative assessment of nodule size all (n = 13) except 1 patient with a mean nodule size less than 0.6 mm had CSPH.

In a subsequent study performed in 168 patients with compensated cirrhosis who had a liver biopsy, septal thickness was an independent predictor of the development of clinical decompensation.[62] Fibrosis area was not evaluated in this study.

Histologic Classification of Cirrhosis

In summary, nodule size, septal width, and fibrosis area are the most important histologic factors that correlate with disease severity in cirrhosis. The question that arises is which of, and how, these features should be incorporated into a pathologic subclassification of cirrhosis that would be easy to assess in order to have widespread applicability.

Studies suggest that architectural features like nodule size, septal width, or other architectural features (eg, contours of the nodules) are better assessed subjectively on routine histopathology by an experienced pathologist, preferably using a special stain to highlight the collagen, most often a trichrome stain, and that their quantitation using image analysis may be less reliable.[60] Although the percentage of biopsy area occupied by fibrous tissue can only be estimated crudely by routine histopathology, requiring a more precise estimation by quantitative morphometric analysis using digital images,[59,60,63,70,71] pathologists should easily be able to differentiate cases in which less than 10% (one-tenth of the area) of the liver biopsy is occupied by fibrous tissue from cases in which greater than 30% (one-third of the area) of the liver biopsy is occupied by fibrosis, numbers that can serve as a rough cutoffs to differentiate patients with and without CSPH.

A proposed classification of cirrhosis based on nodule, size, septal width, and fibrosis thickness area is shown in **Table 1** and this is compared with the Laennec classification.[64] The proposed classification can easily be incorporated into 2 of the most commonly used systems to stage chronic liver disease, the Batts and Ludwig and the METAVIR systems. Their stage 4 (cirrhotic stage) can be further subdivided into 4a, 4b, and 4c. Each parameter can be scored as 1 to 3:

- Thin septa = 1
- Intermediate septa = 2
- Thick septa = 4
- Large nodules = 1
- Mixed nodules = 2
- Small nodules = 3

In combining total scores:

- A score less than 4 implies mild cirrhosis (4a)
- A score of 4 implies moderate cirrhosis (4b)
- A score greater than 4 implies severe cirrhosis (4c), as shown in **Table 2**.

Thus the biopsies with large nodules and septa that are not thick would be classified as mild (early) cirrhosis (stage 4a) and all others with a mixture of nodules and varying septal width as intermediate (4b). Even within the group of severe cirrhosis (4c), presence of small nodules combined with wide septa represents the worst group because the associated HVPG is likely to be greater than 20 mm Hg. The amount of fibrosis would represent an independent parameter; with mild cirrhosis it would tend to be less than 10%, whereas it would be greater than 30% with severe cirrhosis. Assessment of fibrosis area could either be done crudely based on subjective assessment of liver biopsies, or more accurately via morphometric analysis. Further work to introduce the fibrosis area into the scoring system mentioned earlier is needed.

PRACTICAL ISSUES AND FUTURE DIRECTION

The proposed classification is considered a work in progress. There are several practical issues that need to be refined in future studies. This classification needs to be validated to become fully accepted in clinical practice and for research trials. Although the three histologic stages correlate well with disease severity and progression, their correlation with specific clinical features, as outlined in **Table 2**, needs to be studied better and cutoffs for each stage may need to be refined. The classification also needs to be tested for interobserver and intraobserver variability. The original studies largely evaluated cirrhosis caused by viral hepatitis and alcohol, and the system needs to be tested for other causes, especially nonalcoholic steatohepatitis. The impact of sample size, fragmented specimens, and sampling error needs to be investigated, although the original studies show that the parameters were assessed reliably in biopsies that were barely adequate in size (about 1 cm long). It is anticipated that central sclerosis, sinusoidal fibrosis, and capillarization of sinusoidal fibrosis have an important impact on liver dysfunction and their relative significance in a scoring system also needs to tested in future studies.

REFERENCES

1. Bedossa P, Paradis V. Liver extracellular matrix in health and disease. J Pathol 2003;200:504–15.
2. Anthony PP, Ishak KG, Nayak NC, et al. The morphology of cirrhosis. Recommendations on definition, nomenclature, and classification by a working group sponsored by the World Health Organization. J Clin Pathol 1978;31:395–414.
3. Ratziu V, Voiculescu M, Poynard T. Touching some firm ground in the epidemiology of NASH. J Hepatol 2012;56:23–5.
4. Fattovich G, Giustina G, Degos F, et al. Morbidity and mortality in compensated cirrhosis type C: a retrospective follow-up study of 384 patients. Gastroenterology 1997;112:463–72.
5. Bataller R, Brenner DA. Liver fibrosis. J Clin Invest 2005;115:209–18.
6. Friedman SL, Bansal MB. Reversal of hepatic fibrosis – fact or fantasy? Hepatology 2006;43:S82–8.
7. Perez-Tamayo R. Cirrhosis of the liver: a reversible disease? Pathol Annu 1979;14(Pt 2):183–213.

8. Wanless IR, Nakashima E, Sherman M. Regression of human cirrhosis. Morphologic features and the genesis of incomplete septal cirrhosis. Arch Pathol Lab Med 2000;124:1599–607.

9. Serpaggi J, Carnot F, Nalpas B, et al. Direct and indirect evidence for the reversibility of cirrhosis. Hum Pathol 2006;37:1519–26.

10. Reichard O, Glaumann H, Fryden A, et al. Long-term follow-up of chronic hepatitis C patients with sustained virological response to alpha-interferon. J Hepatol 1999;30:783–7.

11. Shiratori Y, Imazeki F, Moriyama M, et al. Histologic improvement of fibrosis in patients with hepatitis C who have sustained response to interferon therapy. Ann Intern Med 2000;132:517–24.

12. George SL, Bacon BR, Brunt EM, et al. Clinical, virologic, histologic, and biochemical outcomes after successful HCV therapy: a 5-year follow-up of 150 patients. Hepatology 2009;49:729–38.

13. D'Ambrosio R, Aghemo A, Rumi MG, et al. Histological findings among HCV cirrhotic patients who achieved a SVR: a morphometric and immunohistochemical study. Hepatology 2011;54:1229A.

14. Poynard T, McHutchison J, Manns M, et al. Impact of pegylated interferon alfa-2b and ribavirin on liver fibrosis in patients with chronic hepatitis C. Gastroenterology 2002;122:1303–13.

15. Dienstag JL, Goldin RD, Heathcote EJ, et al. Histological outcome during long-term lamivudine therapy. Gastroenterology 2003;124:105–17.

16. Chang TT, Liaw YF, Wu SS, et al. Long-term entecavir therapy results in the reversal of fibrosis/cirrhosis and continued histological improvement in patients with chronic hepatitis B. Hepatology 2010;52:886–93.

17. Fauerholdt L, Schlichting P, Christensen E, et al. Conversion of micronodular cirrhosis into macronodular cirrhosis. Hepatology 1983;3:928–31.

18. Czaja AJ, Carpenter HA. Decreased fibrosis during corticosteroid therapy of autoimmune hepatitis. J Hepatol 2004;40:646–52.

19. Cotler SJ, Jakate S, Jensen DM. Resolution of cirrhosis in autoimmune hepatitis with corticosteroid therapy. J Clin Gastroenterol 2001;32:428–30.

20. Niederau C, Fischer R, Purschel A, et al. Long-term survival in patients with hereditary hemochromatosis. Gastroenterology 1996;110:1107–19.

21. Hammel P, Couvelard A, O'Toole D, et al. Regression of liver fibrosis after biliary drainage in patients with chronic pancreatitis and stenosis of the common bile duct. N Engl J Med 2001;344:418–23.

22. Chavez-Tapia NC, Tellez-Avila FI, Barrientos-Gutierrez T, et al. Bariatric surgery for non-alcoholic steatohepatitis in obese patients. Cochrane Database Syst Rev 2010;(1). CD007340.

23. Schuppan D, Pinzani M. Anti-fibrotic therapy: lost in translation? J Hepatol 2012;56(Suppl 1):S66–74.

24. Bedossa P, Dargere D, Paradis V. Sampling variability of liver fibrosis in chronic hepatitis C. Hepatology 2003;38:1449–57.

25. Regev A, Berho M, Jeffers LJ, et al. Sampling error and intraobserver variation in liver biopsy in patients with chronic HCV infection. Am J Gastroenterol 2002;97:2614–8.

26. Knodell RG, Ishak KG, Black WC, et al. Formulation and application of a numerical scoring system for assessing histological activity in asymptomatic chronic active hepatitis. Hepatology 1981;1:431–5.

27. Bedossa P, Poynard T. An algorithm for the grading of activity in chronic hepatitis C. The METAVIR Cooperative Study Group. Hepatology 1996;24:289–93.

28. Hennes EM, Zeniya M, Czaja AJ, et al. Simplified criteria for the diagnosis of autoimmune hepatitis. Hepatology 2008;48:169–76.

29. Wong GL, Yiu KK, Wong VW, et al. Meta-analysis: reduction in hepatic events following interferon-alfa therapy of chronic hepatitis B. Aliment Pharmacol Ther 2010;32:1059–68.

30. Mallet V, Gilgenkrantz H, Serpaggi J, et al. Brief communication: the relationship of regression of cirrhosis to outcome in chronic hepatitis C. Ann Intern Med 2008;149:399–403.

31. Arthur MJ. Collagenases and liver fibrosis. J Hepatol 1995;22:43–8.

32. Bataller R, Gabele E, Parsons CJ, et al. Systemic infusion of angiotensin II exacerbates liver fibrosis in bile duct-ligated rats. Hepatology 2005;41:1046–55.

33. Theret N, Musso O, L'Helgoualc'h A, et al. Activation of matrix metalloproteinase-2 from hepatic stellate cells requires interactions with hepatocytes. Am J Pathol 1997;150:51–8.

34. Uchinami H, Seki E, Brenner DA, et al. Loss of MMP 13 attenuates murine hepatic injury and fibrosis during cholestasis. Hepatology 2006;44:420–9.

35. Iredale JP. Hepatic stellate cell behavior during resolution of liver injury. Semin Liver Dis 2001;21:427–36.

36. Benyon RC, Iredale JP, Goddard S, et al. Expression of tissue inhibitor of metalloproteinases 1 and 2 is increased in fibrotic human liver. Gastroenterology 1996;110:821–31.

37. Geerts A. History, heterogeneity, developmental biology, and functions of quiescent hepatic stellate cells. Semin Liver Dis 2001;21:311–35.

38. de Leeuw AM, McCarthy SP, Geerts A, et al. Purified rat liver fat-storing cells in culture divide and contain collagen. Hepatology 1984;4:392–403.

39. Saile B, Knittel T, Matthes N, et al. CD95/CD95L-mediated apoptosis of the hepatic stellate cell. A mechanism terminating uncontrolled hepatic stellate cell proliferation during hepatic tissue repair. Am J Pathol 1997;151:1265–72.

40. Iredale JP, Benyon RC, Pickering J, et al. Mechanisms of spontaneous resolution of rat liver fibrosis.

Hepatic stellate cell apoptosis and reduced hepatic expression of metalloproteinase inhibitors. J Clin Invest 1998;102:538–49.

41. Gaca MD, Zhou X, Issa R, et al. Basement membrane-like matrix inhibits proliferation and collagen synthesis by activated rat hepatic stellate cells: evidence for matrix-dependent deactivation of stellate cells. Matrix Biol 2003;22:229–39.

42. Taimr P, Higuchi H, Kocova E, et al. Activated stellate cells express the TRAIL receptor-2/death receptor-5 and undergo TRAIL-mediated apoptosis. Hepatology 2003;37:87–95.

43. Issa R, Zhou X, Constandinou CM, et al. Spontaneous recovery from micronodular cirrhosis: evidence for incomplete resolution associated with matrix cross-linking. Gastroenterology 2004;126:1795–808.

44. Rudolph KL, Chang S, Millard M, et al. Inhibition of experimental liver cirrhosis in mice by telomerase gene delivery. Science 2000;287:1253–8.

45. Paradis V, Youssef N, Dargere D, et al. Replicative senescence in normal liver, chronic hepatitis C, and hepatocellular carcinomas. Hum Pathol 2001;32:327–32.

46. Kweon YO, Goodman ZD, Dienstag JL, et al. Decreasing fibrogenesis: an immunohistochemical study of paired liver biopsies following lamivudine therapy for chronic hepatitis B. J Hepatol 2001;35:749–55.

47. Hytiroglou P, Snover DC, Alves V, et al. Beyond "cirrhosis": a proposal from the International Liver Pathology Study Group. Am J Clin Pathol 2012;137:5–9.

48. Garcia-Tsao G, Friedman S, Iredale J, et al. Now there are many (stages) where before there was one: in search of a pathophysiological classification of cirrhosis. Hepatology 2010;51:1445–9.

49. Ripoll C, Groszmann R, Garcia-Tsao G, et al. Hepatic venous pressure gradient predicts clinical decompensation in patients with compensated cirrhosis. Gastroenterology 2007;133:481–8.

50. Garcia-Tsao G, Groszmann RJ, Fisher RL, et al. Portal pressure, presence of gastroesophageal varices and variceal bleeding. Hepatology 1985;5:419–24.

51. Morali GA, Sniderman KW, Deitel KM, et al. Is sinusoidal portal hypertension a necessary factor for the development of hepatic ascites? J Hepatol 1992;16:249–50.

52. Blasco A, Forns X, Carrion JA, et al. Hepatic venous pressure gradient identifies patients at risk of severe hepatitis C recurrence after liver transplantation. Hepatology 2006;43:492–9.

53. Garcia-Pagan JC, Bosch J. Monitoring of HVPG during pharmacological therapy: evidence in favor of the prognostic value of a 20% reduction. Hepatology 2004;39:1746–7 [author reply: 1747].

54. Ripoll C, Groszmann RJ, Garcia-Tsao G, et al. Hepatic venous pressure gradient predicts development of hepatocellular carcinoma independently of severity of cirrhosis. J Hepatol 2009;50:923–8.

55. Saleh HA, Abu-Rashed AH. Liver biopsy remains the gold standard for evaluation of chronic hepatitis and fibrosis. J Gastrointestin Liver Dis 2007;16:425–6.

56. Madan K. Is liver biopsy still the gold standard for diagnosing liver fibrosis? Trop Gastroenterol 2011;32:253–5.

57. Carrion JA, Navasa M, Bosch J, et al. Transient elastography for diagnosis of advanced fibrosis and portal hypertension in patients with hepatitis C recurrence after liver transplantation. Liver Transpl 2006;12:1791–8.

58. Berg T, Sarrazin C, Hinrichsen H, et al. Does noninvasive staging of fibrosis challenge liver biopsy as a gold standard in chronic hepatitis C? Hepatology 2004;39:1456–7 [author reply: 1457–8].

59. Calvaruso V, Burroughs AK, Standish R, et al. Computer-assisted image analysis of liver collagen: relationship to Ishak scoring and hepatic venous pressure gradient. Hepatology 2009;49:1236–44.

60. Sethasine S, Jain D, Groszmann RJ, et al. Quantitative histological-hemodynamic correlations in cirrhosis. Hepatology 2012;55:1146–53.

61. Kumar M, Sakhuja P, Kumar A, et al. Histological subclassification of cirrhosis based on histological-haemodynamic correlation. Aliment Pharmacol Ther 2008;27:771–9.

62. Sreenivasan P, Inayat I, Deng Y, et al. Histological-clinical correlation in cirrhosis-validation of a histological classification of the severity of cirrhosis. Hepatology 2007;46(Suppl 1):579A.

63. Goodman ZD, Stoddard AM, Bonkovsky HL, et al. Fibrosis progression in chronic hepatitis C: morphometric image analysis in the HALT-C trial. Hepatology 2009;50:1738–49.

64. Nagula S, Jain D, Groszmann RJ, et al. Histological-hemodynamic correlation in cirrhosis-a histological classification of the severity of cirrhosis. J Hepatol 2006;44:111–7.

65. Wanless IR, Sweeney G, Dhillon AP, et al. Lack of progressive hepatic fibrosis during long-term therapy with deferiprone in subjects with transfusion-dependent beta-thalassemia. Blood 2002;100:1566–9.

66. Kutami R, Girgrah N, Wanless IR, et al. The Laennec grading system for assessment of hepatic fibrosis: validation by correlation with wedged hepatic vein pressure and clinical features. Hepatology 2000;32:407A.

67. D'Amico G, Garcia-Tsao G, Pagliaro L. Natural history and prognostic indicators of survival in cirrhosis: a systematic review of 118 studies. J Hepatol 2006;44:217–31.

68. Kim MY, Cho MY, Baik SK, et al. Histological sub-classification of cirrhosis using the Laennec fibrosis scoring system correlates with clinical stage and grade of portal hypertension. J Hepatol 2011;55: 1004–9.

69. Xu B, Broome U, Uzunel M, et al. Capillarization of hepatic sinusoid by liver endothelial cell-reactive autoantibodies in patients with cirrhosis and chronic hepatitis. Am J Pathol 2003;163:1275–89.

70. Masseroli M, Caballero T, O'Valle F, et al. Automatic quantification of liver fibrosis: design and validation of a new image analysis method: comparison with semi-quantitative indexes of fibrosis. J Hepatol 2000;32:453–64.

71. Goodman ZD, Becker RL Jr, Pockros PJ, et al. Progression of fibrosis in advanced chronic hepatitis C: evaluation by morphometric image analysis. Hepatology 2007;45:886–94.

Hepatocellular Adenomas
WHO Classification and Immunohistochemical Workup

Valérie Paradis, MD, PhD[a,b,*]

KEYWORDS

• Hepatocellular adenoma • HCA • WHO classification • Hepatocellular carcinoma

ABSTRACT

This review discusses the various subtypes of hepatocellular adenomas (HCAs), their diagnosis, and management. HCAs are benign tumors, mostly seen in young women in a normal background liver. Recent advances in understanding HCA pathogenesis and molecular alterations led to recognition of different subtypes, now included in the WHO classification. Complications include hemorrhage and rarely malignant transformation into hepatocellular carcinoma. Diagnosis and differentiation are challenging, requiring careful attention to clinical setting, histology, and immuostaining profile. Risk of complications varies depending on the HCA; hence, subtyping has clinical significance and is performed based on morphology and use of selected immunohistochemical markers.

Key Features

- Hepatocellular carcinoma is a rare, benign liver tumor strongly associated with oral contraceptive pill use in women and androgen steroid therapy in men.
- Most HCAs develop in a noncirrhotic liver, often without any obvious liver pathology.
- The 3 main subtypes of HCA include the following:
  - Steatotic (30%–40%)
  - Telangiectatic/inflammatory
  - β-catenin activated (10%)
- Subtyping of HCA has clinical significance and can be performed based on morphology and use of selected immunohistochemical markers.

INTRODUCTION

Hepatocellular adenomas (HCAs) are benign hepatocellular tumors, mostly seen in young women usually in a normal background liver. Potential complications include hemorrhage and rarely malignant transformation into hepatocellular carcinoma (HCC). Their diagnosis and differentiation from other benign hepatocellular lesions and well-differentiated HCC remains challenging, especially on needle biopsies.

In the past decade, there have been significant advances in the pathogenesis and molecular alterations in HCA, leading to a comprehensive classification with different subtypes. Accordingly, new guidelines, in terms of diagnosis, prognosis, and therapy, have been proposed. Diagnostic criteria based on magnetic resonance imaging (MRI), for identification of the main HCA subtypes have also been developed. This has also led to a more refined approach to a biopsy diagnosis of benign hepatocellular tumors.

EPIDEMIOLOGIC AND CLINICAL DATA

HCA is a rare, benign liver tumor strongly associated with oral contraceptive pill (OCP) use in

a Pathology Department, Beaujon Hospital, 100 bvd du Général Leclerc, Clichy Cedex 92118, France; b INSERM U773, Faculté de Médecine Xavier Bichat, 16 rue Henri Huchart Paris 75018, France
* Pathology Department, Beaujon Hospital, 100 bu du Général Leclerc, Clichy Cedex 92118, France.
E-mail address: vparadis@teaser.fr

Surgical Pathology 6 (2013) 311–331
http://dx.doi.org/10.1016/j.path.2013.03.008
1875-9181/13/$ – see front matter © 2013 Elsevier Inc. All rights reserved.

women and androgen steroid therapy in men.[1–3] Indeed, its incidence increases from 0.1 per year per 100,000 in non-OCP users to 3 to 4 per 100,000 in long-term OCP users. The other recognized risk factors include hereditary metabolic diseases, such as glycogenosis (type 1 or 3), galactosemia, hepatic iron overload related to beta-thalassemia, and maturity-onset diabetes of the young type 3 (MODY3).[4–6] More recently, metabolic syndrome (MS), especially obesity, has been identified as a new risk factor that is associated with specific HCA subtypes.[7–9]

Clinically, compared with focal nodular hyperplasia (FNH), HCA is more often associated with symptoms and/or liver function test abnormalities. These include abdominal pain and intraperitoneal hemorrhage associated with tumor rupture. Alfafetoprotein (AFP) is commonly in the normal range and its elevation may be suggestive of an underlying HCC. HCA may be single or multiple, and in cases of more than 10 HCAs, the diagnosis of liver adenomatosis is arbitrarily accepted.[10] Patients with multiple HCAs are predominantly women, and have similar imaging features and risk of complications; however, the use of OCPs appears to be less prevalent. Except for the number of lesions, no difference is observed between imaging features of adenomatosis and solitary HCA, and risk of complications is similar to that in patients with solitary HCA, and is not influenced by the number of tumors.

FROM PATHOLOGY TO MOLECULAR FINDINGS: THE PATHOMOLECULAR CLASSIFICATION OF HCA

Macroscopically, HCAs are usually

- Well-defined tumors of varying sizes, that range from microscopic to 30 cm
- Can be pedunculated
- May have large subcapsular vessels on their surface

On cut sections, the tumor may be homogeneous with a fleshy appearance ranging in color from white to brown, or yellow. Some are heterogeneous, especially the large ones, largely due to areas of necrosis and/or hemorrhage. Importantly, most HCAs develop in a noncirrhotic liver, often without any obvious liver pathology.

Histologically, HCA is characterized by

- Proliferation of benign hepatocytes arranged in regular plates of 1 or 2 cells thick.
- No presence of residual portal tracts, but small thin and unpaired vessels are observed throughout the tumor.

- Rare ductules can be seen, especially with cytokeratin 7 or 19.
- Tumoral hepatocytes may appear normal, clear (increased glycogen), steatotic (fat storing), or pigmented.
- A certain degree of nuclear irregularity and slightly increased nucleo-cytoplasm, especially in patients who have taken steroids for many years; however, presence of obvious dysplasia should raise a serious concern for HCC. In that context, differentiation from HCC requires careful examination of the architectural pattern and additional immunohistochemical markers.

Based on genotype-phenotype correlations, a pathomolecular classification of HCA has been elaborated, defining several distinct subtypes.[11] Given the high concordance among morphology, immunophenotype, and genotype, HCA subtyping can be done in routine clinical practice with selected immunohistochemical stains.[12]

Steatotic HCA

Steatotic HCAs represent a homogeneous group of tumors composed of steatotic hepatocytes without significant inflammation or cellular atypia. This subtype accounts for approximately 40% of HCAs, is the most common phenotype observed in liver adenomatosis, and is usually less prone to severe complications, especially malignant transformation to HCC.[13] Genetically, these HCAs display biallelic mutations of hepatocyte nuclear factor 1α (HNF1α).[14] HNF1α mutations are somatic in 90% of cases. Patients with inherited mutation in one allele of HNF1α may develop MODY3 and are predisposed to develop HCA, when the second allele is inactivated in hepatocytes by somatic mutation or chromosomal deletion.[13] As Liver Fatty Acid Binding Protein (LFABP) is positively regulated by HNF1α, its tissue expression may serve as a relevant surrogate marker of HNF1α inactivation. Thus, HNF1α-mutated HCAs are characterized by the absence of LFABP expression in tumoral cells, contrasting with a constitutive positive expression in nontumoral hepatocytes (Fig. 1).[12] Although identification of steatotic LFABP-negative HCA is theoretically easy, either on imaging or histology, in practice problems arise as some tumors have less steatosis. Indeed, in the seminal series, only 36% of LFAPB-negative HCAs displayed extensive steatosis (defined as greater than 60%), whereas 37% of lesions contained less than 30% steatosis.[12] Therefore, immunohistochemistry demonstrating the absence of LFABP expression in the tumor cells could be valuable.

Fig. 1. Steatotic LFABP-negative hepatocellular adenoma. (*A*) Macroscopic view of a well-limited, yellow-tan lesion. (*B*) Tumor is nonencapsulated, with slightly lobulated contours, developed in a non-steatotic liver parenchyma (hematoxylin and eosin [H&E] staining, ×100).

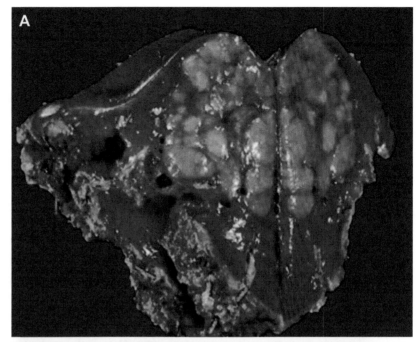

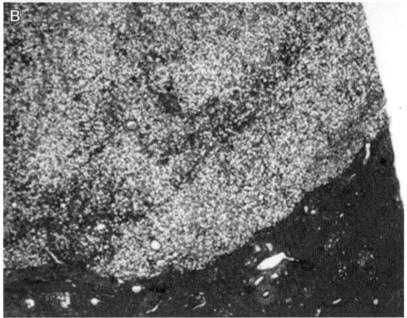

Telangiectatic/Inflammatory Subtype

The telangiectatic/inflammatory (Tel/Inf) HCAs mainly correspond to the initially so-called "telangiectatic form of FNH," described by Wanless and colleagues.[15] Their recognition as HCAs came from molecular studies showing their clonal nature and association with a specific molecular profile related to angiopoietins (ANGPT1 and 2), molecules involved in vascular remodeling. The *ANGPT1:ANGPT2* mRNA ratio in Tel/Inf HCA is close to 1, whereas FNH shows an increased *ANGPT1:ANGPT2* mRNA ratio.[16] Grossly, Tel/Inf

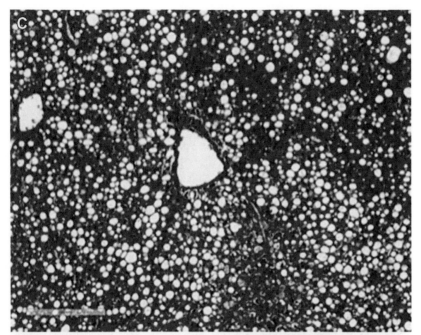

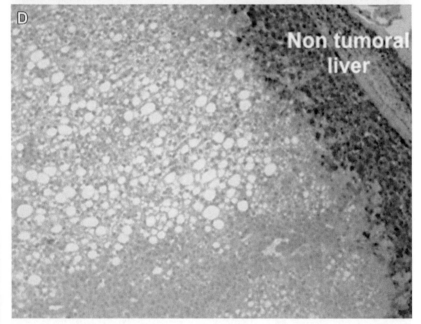

Fig. 1. (*C*) Tumor is made of benign steatotic hepatocytes arranged in regular plates intermingled with small unpaired arteries (H&E staining, ×250). (*D*) LFABP staining (×250) shows absence of expression in tumoral cells compared with nonsteatotic hepatocytes in the adjacent nontumoral liver.

HCAs are well-delineated, unencapsulated tumors with congestion or hemorrhage related to sinusoidal dilation and/or peliotic changes, and lack a central fibrous scar.[15] Microscopically, the hepatocellular proliferation contains few and short fibrous septa around clusters of small vessels, sometimes accompanied by inflammatory infiltrates (mainly composed of lymphocytes and macrophages), and a relatively low ductular reaction (**Fig. 2**). The morphologic features explain their

Fig. 2. Telangiectatic/inflammatory hepatocellular adenoma. (*A*) Macroscopic view shows a well-limited heterogeneous nodule with vascular changes throughout the tumor. (*B*) Tumor is ill defined from the adjacent normal liver, without fibrous capsule (H&E staining, ×100). The *arrows* indicate the interface HCA with the non tumoral liver.

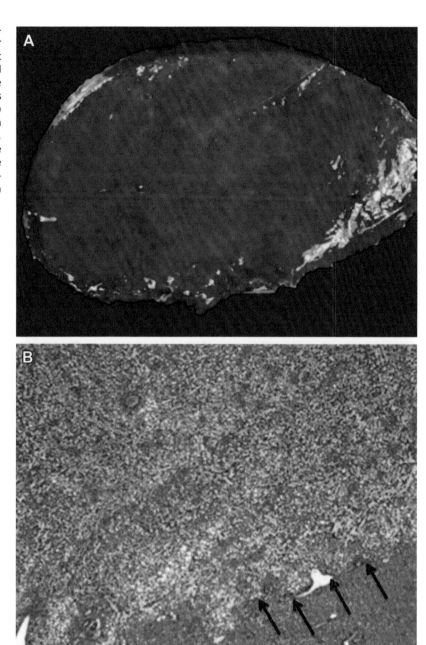

initial recognition as "telangiectatic form of FNH."[15] Notably, steatosis may be observed inside and outside the lesion, with various degrees of intensity.[7] Although commonly observed in women using OCPs for several years, Tel/Inf HCAs have been associated with increased body mass index and a systemic inflammatory syndrome, which includes increased C reactive protein (CRP) or fibrinogen serum levels.[7,17]

Genetically, mutations in the *IL6ST* gene, encoding the signaling coreceptor gp130, and leading to interleukin-6 signaling pathway activation, have been identified in approximately 60% of Tel/Inf HCAs.[18] Gain-of-function somatic mutations in

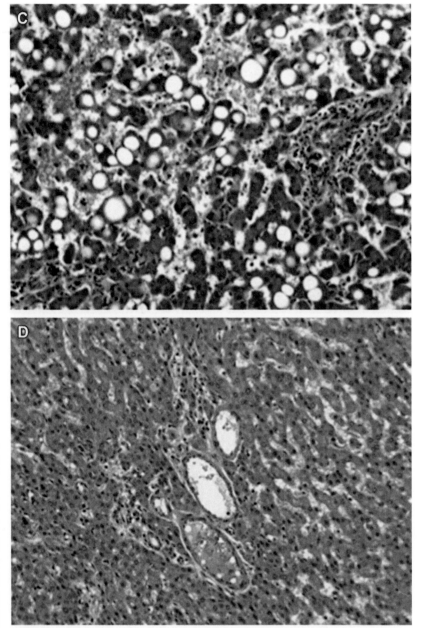

Fig. 2. (C) Proliferation is made of regular hepatocytes, steatotic or not, arranged in thin trabeculae outlined by sinusoidal dilatation. Small arteries are present (H&E staining, ×250). (D) Inside the hepatocellular proliferation, clusters of small arteries are observed, embedded in a small amount of extracellular matrix and few inflammatory cells (H&E staining, ×400).

gp130 may result in the inflammatory phenotype of HCA and explain activation of the acute inflammatory phase reactants observed in tumoral hepatocytes. By immunohistochemistry, Tel/Inf HCAs often express several markers of inflammation, including Serum Amyloid A (SAA) and CRP.[12] **Fig. 3** shows the characteristic immunoprofile of a Tel/Inf HCA, with SAA and LFABP positivity. More recently, somatic mosaic G-protein alpha-subunit (GNAS)-activating mutations have been described in benign hepatocellular tumors, with or without McCune-Albright syndrome, and are characterized by an inflammatory phenotype.[19]

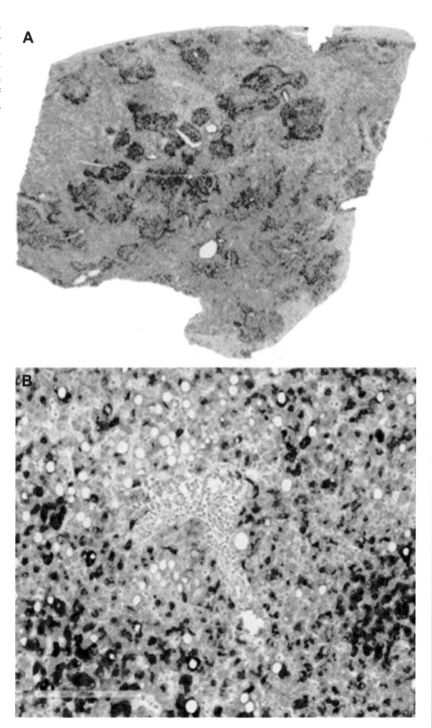

Fig. 3. Telangiectatic/inflammatory hepatocellular adenoma: immunophenotyping. (*A, B*) SAA immunostaining shows diffuse and strong expression of the tumoral hepatocytes (×250).

HCA with Cellular Atypia

The third group of HCAs corresponds to the β-catenin–activated HCAs, which have been initially recognized by the presence of significant cellular atypia of the tumoral hepatocytes.[11] Macroscopically, no specific features are evident, even though they do not display any of the features commonly

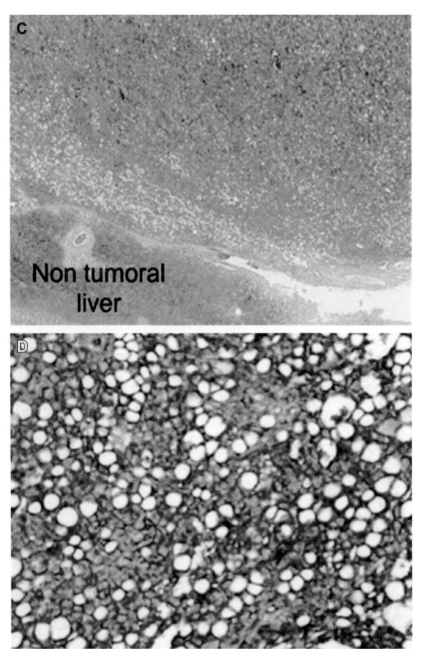

Non tumoral liver

Fig. 3. (*C*) LFABP is expressed both in nontumoral and tumoral hepatocytes (×100). (*D*) Membranous β-catenin is present in tumoral hepatocytes without aberrant cytoplasmic or nuclear positivity (×400).

described in the other subtypes, including vascular or steatotic changes. Usually unique, these HCAs are often observed in male patients and have increased risk of malignant transformation into HCC.[11,20] This subtype accounts for approximately 10% to 15% of all HCAs. Besides the cellular atypia, irregular nuclei, increased nuclear/cytoplasmic ratio, pseudoglandular formations, and cholestasis may be encountered (**Fig. 4**). Differential diagnosis with well-differentiated HCC is the main issue, and extensive sampling of the tumor with careful analysis of the architectural pattern

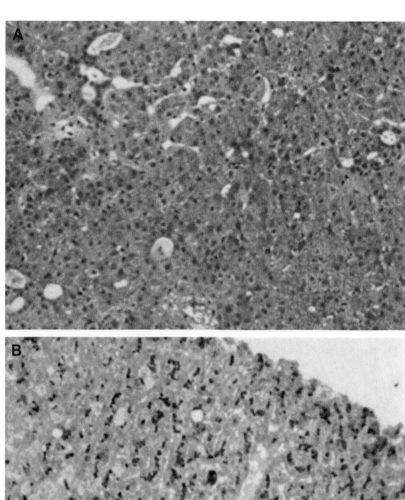

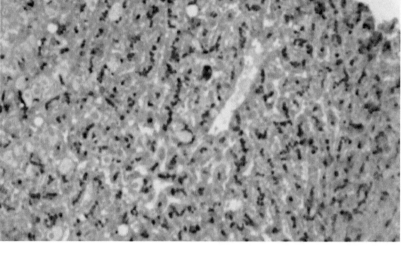

on reticulin stain and surrogate immunophenotypical markers of HCC, including glypican-3, should be performed before calling these HCAs. The diagnosis should be avoided on biopsies and in patients older than 50 years, especially men. Cytogenetic changes similar to HCC have been described in these tumors, suggesting that they may represent very well-differentiated HCC.[21]

In this subtype, activating mutations of *β-catenin* lead to upregulation of its targeted genes, including *GLUL,* encoding glutamine synthetase (GS), and GPR49, encoding orphan nuclear receptor. In these cases, immunohistochemical staining demonstrates a strong and diffuse GS expression in tumoral cells, associated with aberrant nuclear and/or cytoplasmic β-catenin

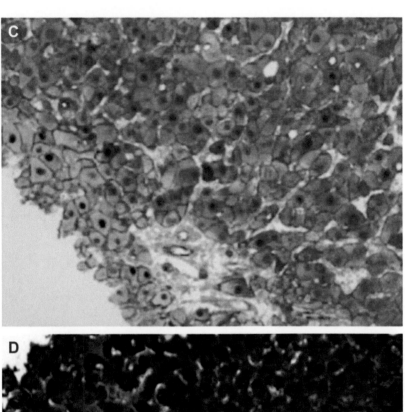

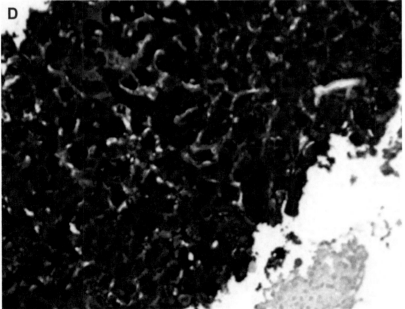

Fig. 4. (C) Extensive cytoplasmic β-catenin positivity with few nuclear staining is observed (×400). *(D)* Strong and diffuse glutamine synthetase staining of the hepatocellular proliferation (×400).

tumoral positivity.[12] Nuclear β-catenin positivity is usually focal and restricted to a few isolated tumoral hepatocytes. Therefore, the GS immunostaining is useful, although diffuse GS positivity does not necessarily imply β-catenin mutation. A case of β-catenin–activated HCA that developed in a man with androgen use is illustrated in **Figs. 4** and **5**. In addition to the HCA with cellular atypia, β-catenin mutations may also be observed in a subset of Tel/Inf HCAs associated with an increased risk of malignant transformation (**Fig. 6**).[12,18,20]

Unclassified HCA

Last, a small group of HCAs (representing 5% to 10%) remains unclassified, as they do not display

Fig. 5. Hepatocellular adenoma associated with androgen use: (A) Macroscopic view of a well-limited centimetric nodule arising in a normal background liver. (B) H&E staining shows a proliferation of hepatocytes arranged in trabeculae intermingled with thin unpaired vessels (H&E staining, ×250).

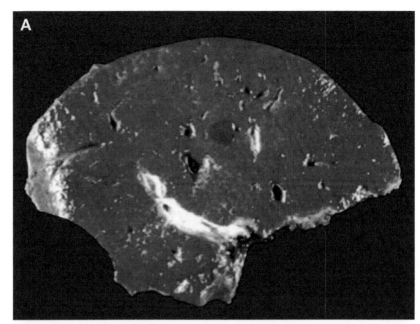

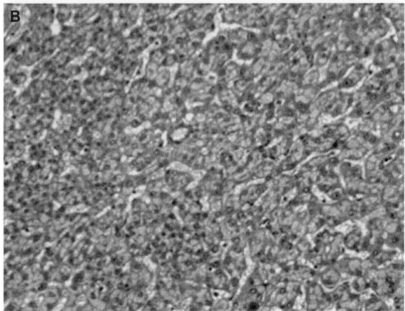

any specific morphologic or genotypical features. Further molecular studies are currently needed for identifying potential genetic characteristics.

Table 1 recapitulates the main genotypical and immunophenotypical characteristics of the different HCA subtypes.

COMPLICATIONS OF HCA

Hemorrhage and Rupture

Compared with FNH, patients with HCA are more likely to present with symptoms, such as abdominal pain, especially when large. In addition, potential serious complications, including spontaneous

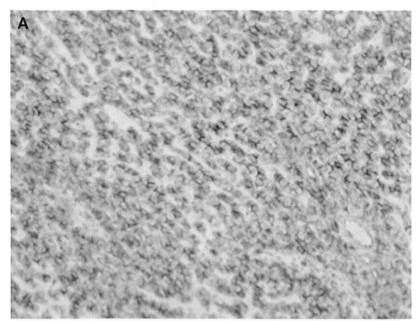

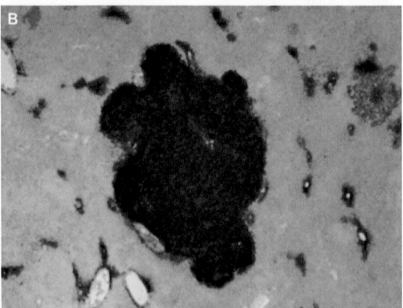

Fig. 6. Hepatocellular adenoma associated with androgen use: immunophenotyping (A) Tumoral hepatocytes display membranous β-catenin expression without aberrant nuclear staining (×250). (B) Glutamine synthetase staining is diffusely and strongly expressed by the tumoral hepatocytes, suggesting the presence of β-catenin activation, even in the absence of the common nuclear β-catenin expression. Note the GS positivity in centrolobular hepatocytes in the adjacent non-tumoral liver (×100).

bleeding, hemorrhage (Fig. 7), and rupture may occur. Such complications occur in 20% to 30% of cases, and symptoms range from abdominal pain to hemodynamic shock, which may require emergent embolization or surgery.[20,22] Several risk factors, including tumor size, Tel/Inf HCA subtype, pregnancy, and recent hormone use,

have been identified to be associated with hemorrhage.[22–24]

Malignant Transformation to HCC

Although rare, transformation of HCA to HCC has been reported. This is of clinical importance and supports potentially aggressive management of

Fig. 6. (C) Reticulin's framework is well preserved (×250). *(D)* Significant cellular atypias (increased nuclear/cytoplasmic ratio and cell pleomorphisms) are observed (H&E staining, ×400).

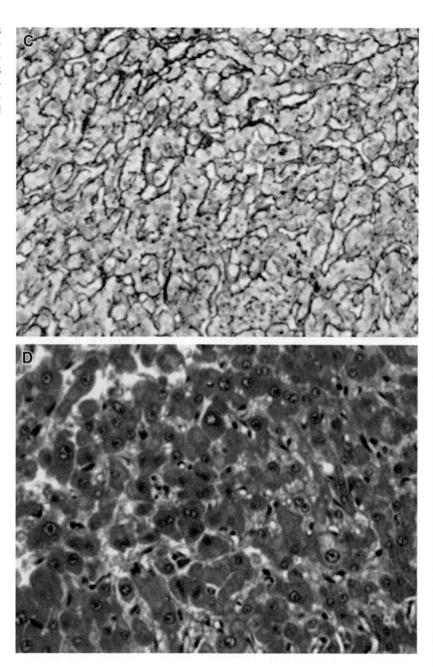

patients with diagnosis of HCA.[20,22–26] A current systematic review, based on the analysis of 1635 HCAs from 157 series and 15 case reports, recently reported an overall frequency of 4.2% of malignant transformation.[27] Progression of HCA to HCC has been suggested based on a variety of evidence. This is possibly best documented in patients with glycogen storage disease type-Ia who are clearly predisposed to multiple HCAs and also HCC. Chromosomal abnormalities have been detected in more than 50% of HCAs analyzed by high-density single nucleotide polymorphism arrays, both in HCAs associated with and without glycogen storage disease Ia.[25,28]

Table 1
Immunophenotypical characteristics of hepatocellular adenomas

Hepatocellular Adenomas Morphologic Diagnosis	Genetic Mutations	LFABP	SAA	β-Catenin	Glutamine Synthetase
Steatotic LFABP negative	HNF1-α	−	−	+ (Membranous)	+ (focal)
Telangiectatic/Inflammatory	*IL6ST*, GNAS	+	+	+ (Membranous)	+ (focal)
Cell atypia	β-catenin	+	−	+ (Nuclear and/or cytoplasmic)	++ (diffuse)
Telangiectatic/Inflammatory + cell atypia	*IL6ST*, GNAS β-catenin	+	+	+ (Nuclear and/or cytoplasmic)	++ (diffuse)
Unclassified HCA	β-catenin	+	−	+ (Membranous)	+ (focal)

Abbreviations: GNAS, mosaic G-protein alpha-subunit; HNF1-α, hepatocyte nuclear factor 1α; IL, interleukin; LFABP, Liver Fatty Acid Binding Protein; SAA, serum amyloid A; (+), positive staining; (−), negative staining.

Molecular studies based on array-based comparative genomic hybridization in a subgroup of atypical hepatocellular neoplasms, defined by either their occurrence in atypical situations (men or women outside the 15–50-year age group) or by atypical morphologic features (small cell changes, prominent acinar architecture, or abnormal trabeculae) showed chromosomal aberrations typically associated with HCC in 53% of these lesions compared with none in typical HCA and 92% in well-differentiated HCC.[29] One could argue that some of these lesions likely represent HCCs that were initially misdiagnosed as HCA. Histologically, rare HCCs have been recognized in a background that resembles an HCA, arising in an otherwise normal liver suggesting a malignant transformation of HCA. HCCs that developed on a preexisting HCA have been described to show 2 main patterns of malignant transformation, one seen macroscopically (mainly encountered in women) and the other seen microscopically (mainly encountered in men).[30] **Figs. 8** and **9** illustrate a macroscopic and microscopic pattern of HCC inside a preexisting HCA, respectively. Most cases of malignant transformation of HCA have been observed at the same time as the diagnosis of HCA, raising a concern that these may represent HCCs with a well-differentiated component; in some cases, however, documented progression to malignancy occurred during clinical follow-up of HCA with time, ranging from 2 to 11 years.[27]

As observed for hemorrhagic complications, malignant progression to HCC is also commonly associated with large size of the tumor, with very few cases (fewer than 5%) described in tumors smaller than 5 cm in diameter.[22,30,31] In addition, several high-risk groups of patients are

recognized, including patients with a history of androgen or anabolic steroid use, male gender, and patients with HCA showing cellular dysplasia usually associated with β-catenin mutations.[3,11,22,30,32] As already noticed, obesity has been clearly associated with an increase in prevalence of HCA, especially for the Tel/Inf subtype.[7,9] In parallel, MS, mainly via obesity and diabetes, is becoming a leading risk factor for HCC.[33,34] In that context, significant numbers of HCCs occur in livers without extensive fibrosis or cirrhosis.[35–37] Some of these tumors may arise from malignant transformation of preexisting HCA.[30,37] For instance, in the surgical series reporting 25 HCAs with transformation to HCC, 6 patients (all men) had MS.[30] Some HCAs never develop complications, either hemorrhage or malignant transformation to HCC.[22,23]

BIOPSY: INDICATIONS AND PERFORMANCE

The general approach of surgical treatment for HCA, compared with watchful waiting for FNH, requires that an accurate diagnosis of HCA. In view of the differences in potential complications, HCA subtyping is considered important. Imaging techniques can provide reliable differentiation between HCA and FNH in most cases, and can help in HCA subtyping. Indeed, several independent studies reported high diagnostic value of imaging, especially MRI, in the characterization of hepatocellular nodules.[38–42] For instance, imaging has been shown to be very reliable for the identification of steatotic LFABP-negative and Tel/Inf subtypes, the 2 most frequent groups of HCA.[39–41] Although additional MRI findings have been proposed for the diagnosis of β-catenin–activated

Fig. 7. Hepatocellular adenomas with hemorrhagic changes. (A) Hepatocellular adenoma showing several small macroscopic hemorrhagic foci. (B) Hepatocellular adenoma with extensive hemorrhagic changes.

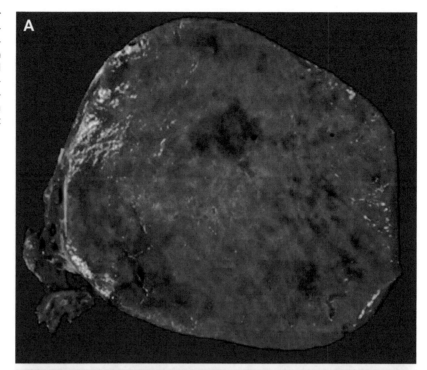

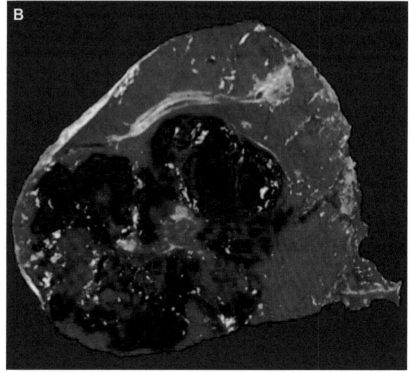

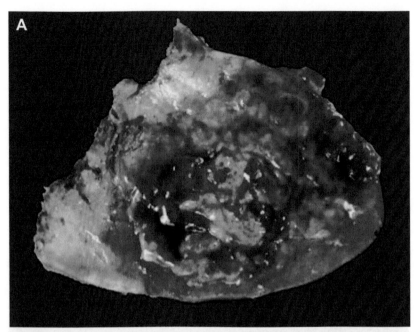

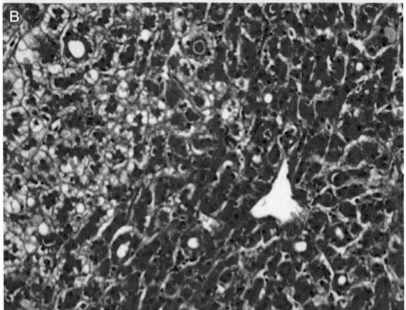

Fig. 8. Hepatocellular carcinoma arising in a pre-existing hepatocellular adenoma (macroscopic pattern). (*A*) Macroscopic view of an ill-defined, heterogeneous tumor, with cholestatic, brown, and necrotic areas developed in a normal background liver. (*B*) Some areas are composed of very well-differentiated hepatocellular proliferation arranged in thin trabeculae, intermingled with unpaired small arteries (H&E staining, ×250).

HCAs, which display the highest risk for malignant transformation, further validation is needed.[41]

Similarly, the characterization of benign hepatocellular nodules on biopsies has improved, mainly due to the application of a variety of immunohistochemical markers that help in the differentiation between FNH and HCA, and enable HCA subtyping.[40,42,43] Because all immunohistochemical stains for HCA subtyping are not widely available, an approach using a limited panel of GS and SAA is discussed in **Table 2**. Even though less crucial than in the context of histologic diagnosis of

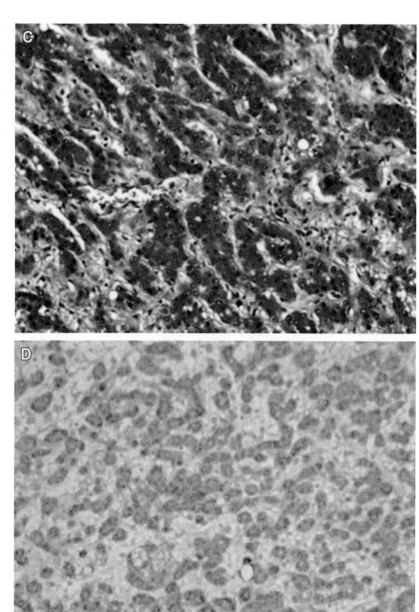

Fig. 8. (*C*) Other areas are malignant, characterized with widened trabeculae of tumoral irregular hepatocytes with extracellular matrix deposits around (H&E staining, ×250). (*D*) Glypican-3 cytoplasmic positivity is observed in malignant hepatocytes (×250).

HCC associated with chronic liver diseases and cirrhosis, biopsy of nontumoral liver may be informative, especially for allowing comparative analysis of the immunophenotypical markers.

MANAGEMENT

In contrast to FNH, active management and further treatment are recommended for HCA because of the potential risk for complications. Management may be individualized from case to case, depending on various parameters, including mainly patient gender, tumor size, and subtype. Indeed, surgical resection is recommended for male patients irrespective of the size of the nodule, and for women if the HCA is larger than 5 cm in diameter.[20,22–24,26,27] As far as HCA subtypes, β-catenin–activated HCAs, mainly because of their high

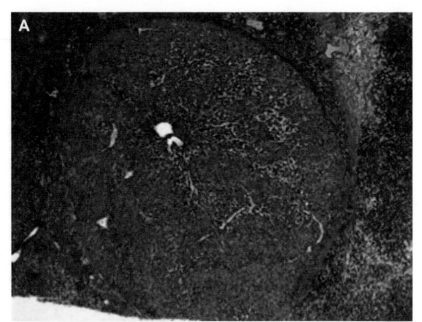

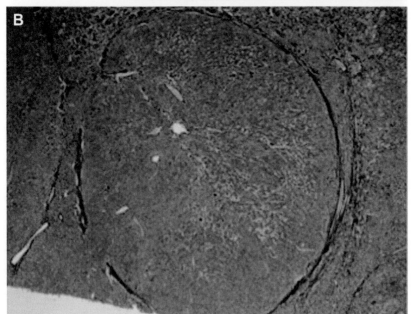

Fig. *9.* Hepatocellular carcinoma arising in a preexisting hepatocellular adenoma (microscopic pattern). (*A*) Low magnification shows microscopic nodular foci of malignant transformation toward hepatocellular carcinoma in an underlying hepatocellular adenoma (H&E staining, ×100). (*B*) Same section with reticulin staining (×100).

propensity to become malignant, and to a lesser extent, Tel/Inf HCAs, because of their higher risk of complications, should be considered for surgical resection. Conversely, small lesions, theoretically associated with a lower risk of complications, can be initially observed. In case of hormonal exposure, cessation of the hormone should be followed by imaging. Importantly,

long-term follow-up of patients with unresected HCAs showed a relative stability for most and even a significant regression in a small proportion of cases after cessation of OCPs.[20,22] **Fig. 10** recapitulates the main criteria taken into account in the therapeutic decision tree.

In conclusion, the significant advances have led to a refined classification of HCAs that has now

Fig. 9. (*C*) β-catenin cytoplasmic expression is focally present in the microscopic malignant foci (×100). (*D*) Glypican-3 staining (×100) demonstrates hepatocellular positivity in the microscopic malignant foci compared with the absence of expression in the surrounding hepatocellular adenoma.

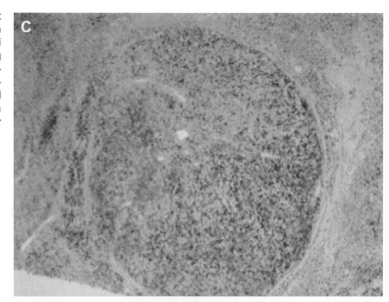

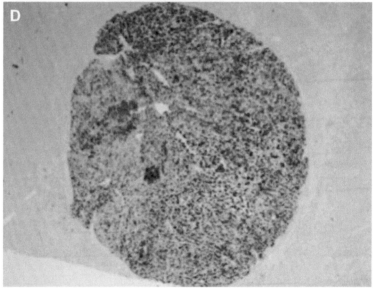

Table 2
Diagnostic approach in hepatocellular lesions using immunohistochemistry for glutamine synthetase (GS) and serum amyloid associated (SAA) protein

Immunohistochemical Results	Diagnosis	Comments
GS: Maplike SAA: negative or patchy positive	FNH	Patchy SAA can be seen in FNH
GS: perivascular or patchy, not maplike SAA: positive	Tel/Inf HCA	Sinusoidal dilatation and inflammation in most cases
GS: strong and diffuse, not maplike SAA: positive	Tel/Inf HCA with β-catenin activation	Sinusoidal dilatation, inflammation and nuclear β-catenin in most cases
GS: strong and diffuse, not maplike SAA: negative	β-catenin–activated HCA or HCC	Carefully review morphology and reticulin for evidence of HCC; cytologic atypia and nuclear β-catenin in most cases
GS: perivascular and patchy, not maplike SAA: negative	HNF1-α-inactivated or unclassified	Prominent steatosis and LFABP loss in HNF1-α-inactivated

Abbreviations: FNH, focal nodular hyperplasia; HCA, hepatocellular adenoma; HCC, hepatocellular carcinoma; HNF1-α, hepatocyte

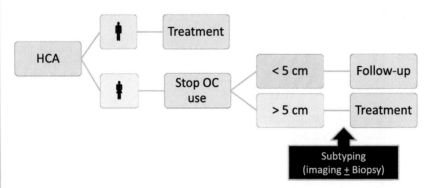

Fig. 10. Management of patients with hepatocellular adenoma. Therapeutic decision depends on gender followed by size and subtyping of the tumor.

been included in the recent World Health Organization classification, which clearly illustrates the major input of combined molecular and morphologic data.

REFERENCES

1. Rooks JB, Ory HW, Ishak KG, et al. Epidemiology of hepatocellular adenomas. The role of oral contraceptive use. JAMA 1979;242:644–8.
2. Coombes GB, Reiser J, Paradinas FJ, et al. An androgen associated hepatic adenoma in a transsexual. Br J Surg 1978;65:869–70.
3. Velazquez I, Alter BP. Androgens and liver tumors: Fanconi's anemia and non-Fanconi's conditions. Am J Hematol 2004;77:257–67.
4. Barthelemes L, Tait IS. Liver cell adenomas and liver cell adenomatosis. HPB (Oxford) 2005;7:186–96.
5. Reznik Y, Dao T, Coutant R, et al. Hepatocyte nuclear factor-1 alpha gene inactivation: cosegregation between liver adenomatosis and diabetes phenotypes in two maturity-onset diabetes of the young (MODY) 3 families. J Clin Endocrinol Metab 2004;89:1476–80.
6. Labrune P, Trioche P, Duvaltier I, et al. Hepatocellular adenomas in glycogen storage disease type I and III: a series of 43 patients and review of the literature. J Pediatr Gastroenterol Nutr 1997;24:276–9.
7. Paradis V, Champault A, Ronot M, et al. Telangiectatic adenomas: an entity associated with increased body mass index and inflammation. Hepatology 2007;46:140–6.
8. Brunt EM, Wolverson MK, Di Bisceglie AM. Benign hepatocellular tumors (adenomatosis) in nonalcoholic steato- hepatitis: a case report. Semin Liver Dis 2005;25:230–6.
9. Bioulac-Sage P, Taouji S, Possenti L, et al. Hepatocellular adenoma subtypes: the impact of overweight and obesity. Liver Int 2012;32:1217–21.
10. Flejou JF, Barges J, Menu Y, et al. Liver adenomatosis: an entity distinct from liver adenoma? Gastroenterology 1985;89:1132–8.
11. Zucman-Rossi J, Jeannot E, Van Nhieu JT, et al. Genotype-phenotype correlation in hepatocellular adenoma: new classification and relationship with HCC. Hepatology 2006;43:515–24.
12. Bioulac-Sage P, Rebouissou S, Thomas C, et al. Hepatocellular adenoma subtype classification using molecular markers and immunohistochemistry. Hepatology 2007;46:740–8.
13. Bacq Y, Jacquemin E, Balabaud C, et al. Familial liver adenomatosis associated with hepatocyte nuclear factor 1 alpha inactivation. Gastroenterology 2003;125:1470–5.
14. Bluteau O, Jeannot E, Bioulac-Sage P, et al. Bi-allellic inactivation of TCF1 in hepatic adenomas. Nat Genet 2002;32:312–5.
15. Wanless IR, Albrecht S, Bilbao J. Multiple focal nodular hyperplasia of the liver associated with vascular malformations of various organs and neoplasia of the brain. Mod Pathol 1989;2:456–62.
16. Paradis V, Benzekri A, Dargère D, et al. Telangiectatic focal nodular hyperplasia: a variant of hepatocellular adenoma. Gastroenterology 2004;126:1323–9.
17. Bioulac-Sage P, Rebouissou S, Sa Cunha A, et al. Clinical morphologic, and molecular features defining so-called telangiectatic focal nodular hyperplasias of the liver. Gastroenterology 2005;128:1211–8.
18. Rebouissou S, Amessou M, Thomas C, et al. Frequent in-frame somatic deletions activate gp130 in inflammatory hepatocellular tumors. Nature 2009;457:2000–4.
19. Nault JC, Fabre M, Couchy G, et al. GNAS activating mutations define a rare subgroup of inflammatory liver tumors characterized by STAT3 activation. J Hepatol 2012;56:184–91.
20. Bioulac-Sage P, Laumonier H, Couchy G, et al. Hepatocellular adenoma management and phenotypic classification: the Bordeaux experience. Hepatology 2009;50:481–9.
21. Evason KJ, Grenert JP, Ferrell LD, et al. Atypical hepatocellular adenoma-like neoplasms with b-catenin activation show cytogenetic alterations similar to

well-differentiated hepatocellular carcinomas. Hum Pathol 2013;44:750–8.

22. Dokmak S, Paradis V, Vilgrain V, et al. A single-center surgical experience of 122 patients with single and multiple hepatocellular adenomas. Gastroenterology 2009;137:1698–705.

23. Deneve JL, Pawlik TM, Cunningham S, et al. Liver cell adenoma: a multicenter analysis of risk factors for rupture and malignancy. Ann Surg Oncol 2009; 16:640–8.

24. van Aalten SM, Witjes CD, de Man RA, et al. Can a decision-making model be justified in the management of hepatocellular adenoma? Liver Int 2012; 32:28–37.

25. Paradis V, Laurent A, Fléjou JF, et al. Evidence for the polyclonal nature of focal nodular hyperplasia of the liver by the study of X chromosome inactivation. Hepatology 1997;26:891–5.

26. Cho SW, Marsh JW, Steel J, et al. Surgical management of hepatocellular adenoma: take it or leave it? Ann Surg Oncol 2008;15:2795–803.

27. Stoot JH, Coelen RJ, de Jong MC, et al. Malignant transformation of hepatocellular adenomas into hepatocellular carcinomas: a systematic review including more than 1600 adenoma cases. HPB (Oxford) 2010;12:509–22.

28. Kishnani PS, Chuang TP, Bali D, et al. Chromosomal and genetic alterations in human hepatocellular adenomas associated with type Ia glycogen storage disease. Hum Mol Genet 2009;18:4781–90.

29. Kakar S, Chen X, Ho C, et al. Chromosomal abnormalities determined by comparative genomic hybridization are helpful in the diagnosis of atypical hepatocellular neoplasms. Histopathology 2009;55:197–205.

30. Farges O, Ferreira N, Dokmak S, et al. Changing trends in malignant transformation of hepatocellular adenoma. Gut 2011;60:85–9.

31. Micchelli ST, Vivekanandan P, Boitnott JK, et al. Malignant transformation of hepatic adenomas. Mod Pathol 2008;21:491–7.

32. Gorayski P, Thompson CH, Subhash HS, et al. Hepatocellular carcinoma associated with recreational anabolic steroid use. Br J Sports Med 2008;42:74–5.

33. Nordenstedt H, White DL, El-Serag HB. The changing pattern of epidemiology in hepatocellular carcinoma. Dig Liver Dis 2010;42:S206–14.

34. Nair S, Mason A, Eason J, et al. Is obesity an independent risk factor for hepatocellular carcinoma in cirrhosis? Hepatology 2002;36:150–5.

35. Guzman G, Brunt EM, Petrovic LM, et al. Does nonalcoholic fatty liver disease predispose patients to hepatocellular carcinoma in the absence of cirrhosis? Arch Pathol Lab Med 2008;132:1761–6.

36. Kawada N, Imanaka K, Kawaguchi T, et al. Hepatocellular carcinoma arising from non-cirrhotic nonalcoholic steatohepatitis. J Gastroenterol 2009;44: 1190–4.

37. Paradis V, Zalinski S, Chelbi E, et al. Hepatocellular carcinomas in patients with metabolic syndrome often develop without significant fibrosis: a pathological analysis. Hepatology 2009;49:851–9.

38. Lewin M, Handra-Luca A, Arrivé L, et al. Liver adenomatosis: classification pf MR imaging features and comparison with pathologic findings. Radiology 2006;241:433–40.

39. Laumonier H, Bioulac-Sage P, Laurent C, et al. Hepatocellular adenomas: magnetic resonance imaging features as a function of molecular pathological classification. Hepatology 2008;48:808–18.

40. Ronot M, Bahrami S, Calderaro J, et al. Hepatocellular adenomas: accuracy of magnetic resonance imaging and liver biopsy in subtype classification. Hepatology 2011;53:1182–91.

41. van Aalten SM, Thomeer MG, Terkivatan T, et al. Hepatocellular adenomas: correlation of MR imaging findings with pathologic subtype classification. Radiology 2011;261:172–81.

42. Ronot M, Paradis V, Duran R, et al. MR findings of steatotic focal nodular hyperplasia and comparison with other fatty tumours. Eur Radiol 2013;23(4): 914–23.

43. Bioulac-Sage P, Cubel G, Taouji S, et al. Immunohistochemical markers on needle biopsies are helpful for the diagnosis of focal nodular hyperplasia and hepatocellular adenoma subtypes. Am J Surg Pathol 2012;36:1691–9.

Diagnostic Approach to Hepatic Mass Lesions and Role of Immunohistochemistry

Esmeralda Celia Marginean, MD[a],*, Allen M. Gown, MD[b],
Dhanpat Jain, MD[c]

KEYWORDS

- Liver mass lesions • Hepatocellular carcinoma • Focal nodular hyperplasia • Hepatic adenoma
- Liver metastatic carcinoma

ABSTRACT

This review provides an overview of various hepatic mass lesions and a practical diagnostic approach, including most recent immunohistochemical stains used in clinical practice. A wide variety of benign and malignant lesions present as hepatic masses, and the differential diagnosis varies. In cirrhotic liver, the commonest malignant tumor is hepatocellular carcinoma (HCC), which needs to be differentiated from macroregenerative nodules, dysplastic nodules, and other tumors. The differential diagnosis of lesions in noncirrhotic liver in younger patients includes hepatic adenoma (HA), focal nodular hyperplasia (FNH), HCC, and other primary hepatic neoplasms and metastases. In older populations, metastases remain the most common mass lesions.

OVERVIEW

In clinical practice, a wide variety of benign and malignant lesions present as hepatic masses and some, if not all, require histologic confirmation. The differential diagnosis varies depending on the age, gender, serum tumor markers, imaging characteristics, and presence of background liver disease, most importantly cirrhosis. From a practical viewpoint, mass lesions could be approached differently in cirrhotic versus noncirrhotic livers. In cirrhotic liver, although any of the other lesions discussed

subsequently may occur, the commonest malignant tumor is hepatocellular carcinoma (HCC), which needs to be differentiated from macroregenerative nodules (MRN), and dysplastic nodules (DN). In this setting, the possibility of an HA or focal nodular hyperplasia (FNH) is less common and even metastases are uncommon. In noncirrhotic liver, especially in patients older than 50 years, the most common mass lesions encountered are metastases; other mass lesions include HCC, FNH, and HA; primary cholangiocarcinoma (CC), mixed HCC-CC. Less common are mesenchymal tumors, such as vascular tumors (hemangioma, epithelioid hemangioendothelioma, and angiosarcoma); angiomyolipoma (AML), and lymphoid neoplasms (Table 1). In children, especially younger than 5 years, the commonly encountered primary hepatic malignancies include hepatoblastoma, mesenchymal hamartoma, and embryonal sarcoma; however, the approach to pediatric neoplasms is different and they are not discussed in this article.

The diagnostic workup of these lesions includes careful evaluation of clinical history, serum tumor markers, imaging findings, and histologic features followed by a judicious immunohistochemical (IHC) panel, especially in biopsies with limited material, and also to avoid unnecessary costs. This review outlines a practical approach to liver mass lesions and describes the frequently used IHC markers in commonly encountered clinical situations, along with their usefulness and limitations.

[a] Department of Pathology, The Ottawa Hospital, Ottawa University, CCW- Room 4251, 501 Smyth Road, Ottawa, Ontario K1H 8L6, Canada; [b] PhenoPath Laboratories, Seattle, WA 98103, USA; [c] Department of Pathology, Yale University School of Medicine, New Haven, CT 06520-8023, USA
* Corresponding author.
E-mail address: cmarginean@toh.on.ca

Surgical Pathology 6 (2013) 333–365
http://dx.doi.org/10.1016/j.path.2013.03.005
1875-9181/13/$ – see front matter © 2013 Published by Elsevier Inc.

Table 1
Most common hepatic mass lesions in cirrhotic and noncirrhotic liver

Cirrhotic Liver	Noncirrhotic Liver
HCC	<u><50 y</u>
MRN	HA
DN	FNH
CC/HCC-CC	HCC
Metastases	Other primary
Other rare primary	tumors of liver
liver tumors	Metastases
	<u>>50 y</u>
	Metastases
	HCC
	FNH
	Other primary
	tumors of liver

MASS LESIONS IN CIRRHOTIC LIVER

MRN

Advances in imaging modalities have led to detection of smaller and smaller nodules in patients with cirrhosis and chronic liver diseases. However, there is considerable confusion regarding their nomenclature and diagnostic criteria, despite attempts at standardization and a consensus approach. The International Consensus Group for Hepatocellular Neoplasia classified nodular lesions in cirrhotic livers into MRN, low-grade DN (LGDN) and high-grade DN (HGDN).[1] They also defined small HCC as all tumors 2 cm or less. The diagnostic criteria for MRN, DN, and early HCC are qualitative, and hence subjective and especially difficult to apply on liver biopsies (Table 2).[2]

Nodules that are larger than 5 mm but lack cytologic or architectural atypia are considered MRN. Nodules with cytologic or architectural dysplasia insufficient for a diagnosis of HCC are considered DN.[1,2]

LGDN

LGDN are often distinct from surrounding liver because of fibrous tissue around the nodule. They show mild increase in cell density and lack cytologic atypia, although they may show large cell changes. Unpaired arteries are sometimes present in small numbers.[1,2] The cell plates display normal thickness and contain portal tracts and central veins. LGDN are difficult to separate from MRN on needle biopsies and the morphologic criteria have proved unreliable and not reproducible.[1,2]

HGDN

HGDN show cytologic atypia, usually small cell change (formerly referred to as small cell dysplasia) and increased cell density, but the

Table 2
Classification of small hepatocellular lesions in cirrhotic liver

Lesion Type		Microscopic Features
Dysplastic foci		Clusters of hepatocytes <1 mm with small cell change
MRN		Regenerative nodules larger than most cirrhotic nodules (>5 mm); contain few portal tracts and 2-cell-thick trabeculae, lined by sinusoids; lacks dysplasia
DN	LGDN	Distinct nodular lesion, mild increase in cell density, may have large cell changes but not architectural atypia; contain few portal tracts
	HGDN	Frank cytologic and architectural atypia, but insufficient to diagnose HCC; increased cell density and focal small cell change; may contain few unpaired arteries; no stromal invasion; CK7/19-positive ductular reaction along the nodule
Small HCC (≤2 cm)	Early HCC	Vaguely nodular lesion, incomplete or absent fibrous capsule, well-differentiated histology, may have focal acinar structures, a few portal tracts, a few unpaired arteries; may contain steatosis; loss of reticulin framework; stromal invasion into portal tracts or fibrous septa; loss of ductular reaction along the nodule
	Progressed HCC	Distinctly nodular lesion; clearly malignant, grade 1 or 2; no portal tracts; pushing growth pattern and fibrous capsule; rarely steatotic as a result of complete neoarterialization; may have appearance of nodule-in-nodule

features are insufficient to clearly diagnose HCC. A few unpaired nontriadal arteries may be seen. Partial sinusoidal capillarization is noted.[3] Pseudoacini are absent or rare. A nodule growing within an HGDN (the nodule-in-nodule appearance) is likely an HCC.[1,2] The most reliable criterion that distinguishes HGDN from early HCC is stromal invasion into portal tracts, fibrous septa, or adjacent parenchyma, but this feature may be absent in biopsies.[1,2] Ductular reaction around nodules is prominent in most cases of MRN and DN, and absent in HCC; it can be highlighted by CK7 or CK19 stains.[4]

HCC

The dogma that any nodule in cirrhotic liver is HCC until proved otherwise still stands. HCC can be classified in small HCC (2 cm or less) and conventional HCC (>2 cm). Small HCC, has been further classified into *early HCC*, with a vaguely nodular appearance, well-differentiated histology, and frequent steatosis; and *progressed HCC*, with distinctly nodular pattern, well-differentiated, or moderately differentiated and often with vascular invasion (Table 2).[1] Progressed HCC can arise de novo, from preexisting HGDN or from an early HCC (giving the gross and radiologic appearance of nodule-in-nodule).[5] At the earliest stage, progressed HCC is 2 cm or less, has a destructive and pushing growth pattern, lacks portal tracts, has a tumor capsule, and shows complete neoarterialization and therefore is usually nonsteatotic. Early HCC has a longer time to recurrence and a higher 5-year survival rate than progressed HCC and hence their separation into distinct categories.[6] The biopsy diagnosis of early HCC is challenging and not entirely reliable, because of sampling errors, and the most reliable criteria are absence of stromal invasion and prominent pseudoacinar differentiation. Therefore, a negative biopsy does not rule out malignancy. Reticulin stain can be useful in this setting, but IHC hepatocytic markers are not useful in this setting. The combination of glypican 3 (GPC3), glutamine synthetase (GS), CD34, and heat shock protein 70 (discussed later in detail) has been advocated, but is seldom diagnostic.

Most nodules greater than 2 cm in cirrhotic liver are HCC and can be diagnosed on contrast-enhanced imaging (computed tomography or magnetic resonance imaging) by the presence of typical hypervascularity in arterial phase and washout in portal venous phase. Biopsy is usually not required in this setting, especially if the serum α-fetoprotein level is also increased, and these nodules are treated by radiofrequency ablation,

transarterial chemoembolization, liver transplantation, or resection, depending on Barcelona Clinic Liver Cancer stage. Biopsy is required only when the imaging is not typical of HCC.[7–10] For tumors between 1 and 2 cm, two concordant radiologic tests are needed for a noninvasive diagnosis of HCC, otherwise biopsy is indicated.[9,11]

Morphologically many tumors, especially well-differentiated to moderately differentiated HCC, do not pose any diagnostic difficulty. Histologically, the tumor cells clearly resemble hepatocytes and show easily identifiable features suggestive of malignancy, which include cytologic atypia, nuclear pleomorphism, thick hepatic cords (>3 cell plates thick), pseudoacini, and loss of reticulin fibers. Cells may have eosinophilic, steatotic, or sometimes clear cytoplasm. A variety of intrahepatocytic inclusions may be seen that include Mallory hyaline, bile, diastase periodic acid Schiff–positive eosinophilic globules, and pale bodies. HCC may show several architectural patterns: trabecular, acinar/pseudoglandular, solid, clear cell, fibrolamellar, and scirrhous type. Well-differentiated to moderately differentiated HCC in a background of cirrhosis usually does not require any confirmation by IHC; however, occasionally one can use HepPar-1 antigen or arginase 1 (Arg1) to confirm hepatocytic differentiation. Reticulin stain can help by delineating the thick trabeculae and loss of reticulin network.

Poorly differentiated HCC (PD-HCC) is easy to recognize as malignant; however, one may need to confirm their hepatocytic nature by IHC to differentiate them from metastases (unusual in cirrhotic liver), CC/mixed tumor, or other rare primary liver tumors (Fig. 1). The markers that are useful in the setting of poorly differentiated tumors are Arg1, HepPar-1, and polyclonal carcinoembryonic antigen (pCEA)/CD10, although HepPar-1 and pCEA have lower sensitivity in PD-HCC. GPC3 can be expressed in a variety of other tumors as well; however because malignancy is not in question in this setting, it is less useful. However, if GPC3 is used, it should be interpreted carefully, although other tumors with GPC expression, like germ cell tumors, mesothelioma, and squamous cell carcinoma, are unusual in the liver and often have distinct morphology.

Also, in the setting of cirrhosis, although FNH or HA can arise, these are extremely rare; these diagnoses should be made with caution, and should be largely restricted to the examination of resection specimens[12–14] or with known predisposing conditions. Recently, HA-like nodules were described in a background of alcoholic cirrhosis.[15] These nodules, unlike HCC, showed strong reactivity for serum amyloid A associated protein

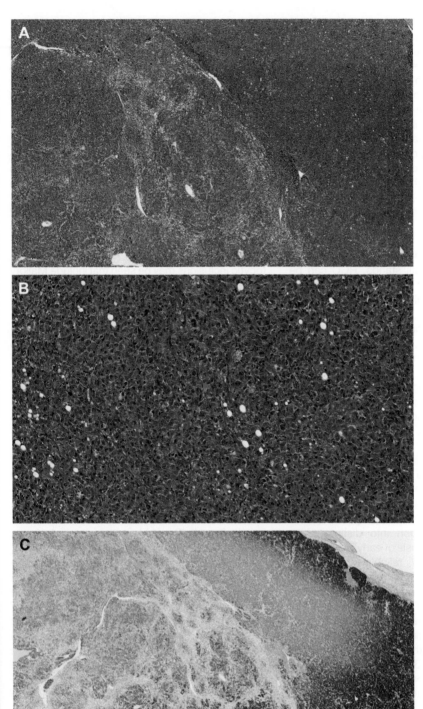

Fig. 1. HCC. (A) Moderately to poorly differentiated HCC (hematoxylin-eosin, original magnification ×20). (B) Moderately to poorly differentiated HCC (hematoxylin-eosin, original magnification ×40). Diffuse cytoplasmic staining of tumor cells with GPC3 (C).

Fig. 1. GS (*D*) at 20×, HepPar1 (*E*) and Arg1 (*F*) at 100×.

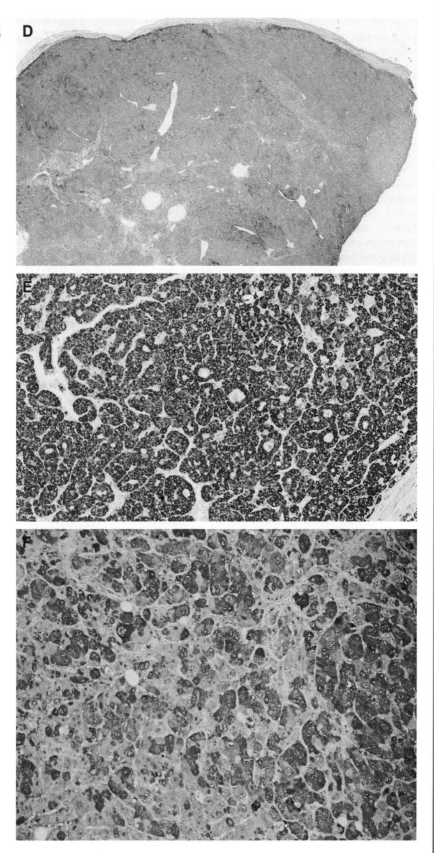

(SAA) and no expression for GS or GPC3 and may be a special, novel type of inflammatory hepatocellular adenomas arising in alcoholic cirrhosis.[15]

HCC Variant: Fibrolamellar HCC

Fibrolamellar hepatocellular carcinoma (FLC) is a distinct variant of HCC, which typically arises in a younger age group, without preexisting cirrhosis, although sometimes they can arise in older patients, or rarely in combination with conventional HCC. The tumor cells are polygonal, large with abundant eosinophilic granular cytoplasm, show conspicuous eosinophilic macronucleoli, and are invested within abundant collagenous stroma, which has a lamellar appearance. Slightly pale eosinophilic, fibrinogen-containing cytoplasmic inclusions (pale bodies) are frequently present.[12,16,17] The diagnosis of FLC can be established on hematoxylin-eosin sections in most cases; however, these tumors have a distinct IHC profile, which can be useful in borderline cases. They are generally positive for HepPar-1, show a typical granular cytoplasmic staining with CD68, and frequently express CK7 and CK19, although there is no evidence of true cholangiolar differentiation.[18]

MASS LESIONS IN NONCIRRHOTIC LIVER

From a practical standpoint, the liver mass lesions can be divided into well-differentiated, clearly hepatocytic tumors (well-differentiated HCC, HA, and FNH); and tumors that are poorly differentiated, clearly malignant, and need confirmation of their hepatocytic lineage.

TUMORS OF HEPATOCYTIC LINEAGE

Hepatic Adenoma

HA is a rare, benign neoplasm that occurs mostly in women and has been associated with oral contraceptive use. It can be single or multiple; the term adenomatosis is appropriate when more than 10 tumors are present.[19] Other causes in women, men, and children include use of anabolic steroids, antiepileptic drugs, vascular disorders (Budd-Chiari syndrome, portal vein shunts, or agenesis), genetic disorders (maturity-onset diabetes of the young type 3 [MODY 3],[20] familial adenomatous polyposis, and Peutz-Jeghers syndrome) and metabolic disorders such as glycogen storage disease.[21,22] During its evolution, HA may remain stable, increase in size, or regress.[23] Transformation into HCC has been reported, mostly in tumors related to androgen or anabolic steroids exposure and in β-catenin–activated HA[23,24]; however, this situation still remains controversial,

because these tumors may be extremely well-differentiated HCC.

Histologically, the neoplasm is sometimes demarcated from adjacent normal liver by a pseudocapsule or compressed liver cords, and is composed of relatively monomorphic hepatocytes, lacks true portal tracts, and shows thin-walled unpaired arteries. Similar to HCC, bile, steatosis, lipofuscin, Dubin-Johnson–like coarsely granular brown pigment, Mallory hyaline, peliosis, and extramedullary hematopoiesis may be seen in HA.[11]

Differentiation of HA from HCC

Distinguishing HA from well-differentiated HCC in a noncirrhotic liver may be difficult, especially in needle biopsies, when sometimes only a diagnosis of well-differentiated hepatocytic neoplasm can be rendered and final diagnosis made only on the resection. As a general guideline, a diagnosis of HA should be offered with extreme caution in patients older than 50 years and men of any age, unless a predisposing cause is known (glycogen storage disease or estrogen/androgen use). Presence of thick hepatic plates (>3 cells), reticulin loss, pseudoglandular differentiation, and small cell change support a diagnosis of HCC. Besides reticulin stain, IHC makers like GPC3, GS, and CD34 can be helpful (Table 3). GPC3 is positive in HCC (Fig. 1), especially moderately to poorly differentiated HCC, and negative in benign liver, HA, and FNH.[17] Although initial reports suggested GPC3 to be expressed in greater than 90% of HCC,[25,26] subsequent experience suggested that in well-differentiated tumors, especially those that are difficult to differentiate from HA or DN/MRN, its positivity decreases to less than 50%.[27] Thus, a positive GPC3 is useful, but a negative GPC3 does not rule out a well-differentiated HCC.

Evidence of diffuse capillarization of sinusoids, most commonly using CD34, supports a diagnosis of HCC; however, it can also be seen in some cases of HA and FNH.[28,29] CD34 normally stains the endothelium of portal vessels, central veins, and a few cells in the inlet of the sinuses. Increasing staining of the periportal and periseptal sinuses can be seen in cirrhotic nodules, FNH, and HA. Thus small nodules, tangential sectioning of nodules or the periseptal areas can mimic diffuse staining of the sinuses, particularly in needle biopsies; hence, caution is warranted in interpreting CD34 stain. One should be skeptical in making a diagnosis of HCC solely based on this stain, although in combination with other findings or markers, it can provide supportive evidence for HCC.

Table 3
Practical IHC panel in the diagnosis of hepatocytic lesions in noncirrhotic liver

Liver Mass Lesion		GPC3	GS	β-catenin (Nuclear)	LFABP	SAA/CRP	CD34
HCC		+	+	−	+	−	+ (diffuse)
HA	HNF1α	−	−	−	−	−	± (focal)
	β-Catenin HA	−	+ (strong, diffuse)	+ (nuclear)	+	−	
	Inflammatory HA	−	−	−	+	+	
	HA, NOS	−	−	−	+	−	
FNH		−	+ (maplike)	−	+	−	± (focal)
Normal liver		−	− (except few hepatocytes in zones 3)	−	+	−	−

Subclassification of hepatic adenoma

Recently, genomic and molecular studies have led to the recognition of several HA subtypes: hepatocyte nuclear factor 1 α (HNF1α)-inactivated, β-catenin–activated, inflammatory, and unclassified HA. This classification was developed by the group in Bordeaux and incorporated in 2010 World Health Organization Tumors of the Digestive System classification. It has been suggested that β-catenin–activated HA carry a high risk of malignant transformation into HCC.[30,31] IHC markers that are used for classification of HA are liver fatty acid binding protein (LFABP), SAA-associated protein, C reactive protein (CRP), β-catenin, and GS (**Table 3**).

HNF1α-inactivated HA Biallelic inactivating mutations in the HNF1α gene occur in 35% to 40% of HA.[21,30–33] HNF1α controls the expression of liver-specific genes, such as β fibrinogen, α₁ antitrypsin, and albumin. Inactivation of HNF1α promotes lipogenesis. Biallelic inactivating HNF1α mutations are somatic in origin, whereas in less than 10% of cases, one mutation is of germline origin, whereas the other is somatic. Patients with germline mutations of HNF1α are younger than those with somatic mutations; they frequently have a family history of liver adenomatosis[34]; and they may have MODY3.[19,21–23,35]

Histologically, these HA are characterized by marked steatosis and lack cytologic atypia or inflammatory infiltrates. They also lack expression of LFABP, in contrast to the nontumoral surrounding liver, which appears homogeneously, although faintly stained (**Fig. 2**).[22] LFABP is a small protein involved in the intracellular transport of long-chain fatty acids in the liver. LFABP is regarded as a sensitive marker for liver cell damage. Furthermore, the downregulation of LFABP may contribute to the fatty phenotype through impaired fatty-acid trafficking.[21,35,36] These tumors also lack expression of SAA, CRP, or nuclear β-catenin, whereas GS shows a normal pericentral pattern.

β-catenin–activated HA Activating β-catenin mutations have been reported in 10% to 15% of all HA[35] and 10% of inflammatory HA.[30] They tend to occur in men and in patients older than 50 years[21,35,36] and histologically are characterized by mild cytologic atypia and acinar pattern. Therefore, these adenomas are difficult to distinguish from well-differentiated HCC, and many believe that these in fact may be well-differentiated HCC. Based on studies from the United States and our own experience, β-catenin–mutated HA are rare if strict histologic and clinical criteria are applied. By IHC, these HA express aberrant nuclear and cytoplasmic β-catenin and are diffusely positive for GS (**Fig. 3**).[21,31]

Inflammatory HA Inflammatory HA account for 40% to 60% of all HA and are associated with activation of the interleukin 6 signaling pathway.[35] This subtype includes most lesions previously called telangiectatic FNH.[31,37] Clinically, these patients often have a high body mass index, a history of alcohol consumption,[21] and may have symptoms of an inflammatory syndrome, including increased serum CRP levels.[31] Morphologically, these tumors show inflammatory infiltrates, composed of lymphocytes, histiocytes, rare plasma cells, and neutrophils, often grouped around thick-walled arteries. Focal ductular reaction (which may not be focal in all cases) similar to FNH is seen around the vessels; however, the typical central scar seen in FNH is absent. The tumors show marked sinusoidal dilatation, rarely peliosis, and hemorrhage. By IHC, they express acute phase inflammatory proteins such as SAA and CRP, with a sharp

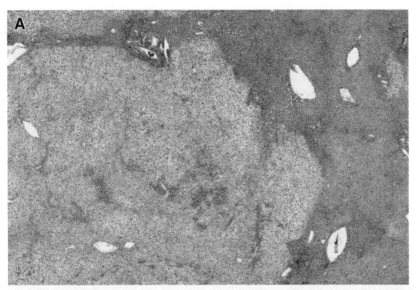

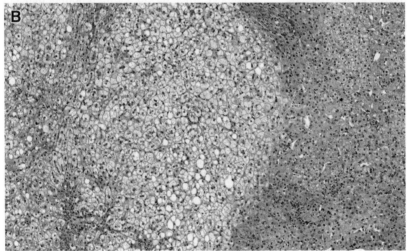

Fig. 2. HNF1α-inactivated HA. (A, B) Relatively well-demarcated, unencapsulated hepatocytic neoplasm, with marked steatosis and no atypia.

demarcation from adjacent nontumoral liver (surrounding liver is often positive, but usually not so strong), as well as LFABP (Fig. 4).[31] They do not show diffuse GS or nuclear β-catenin expression.

HA, unclassified About 5% to 10% of HA fail to show any specific features and remain unclassified.[31] By IHC, they show cytoplasmic LFABP, pericentral GS, and no nuclear β-catenin, SAA, or CRP.

Focal Nodular Hyperplasia

FNH is a common benign lesion that is more common in women, with an estimated prevalence

10 times greater than HA,[23,38] which arises in normal liver in response to a localized hyperperfusion of the liver associated with arterial malformations.[23] Although this lesion is currently believed to be a reactive and hyperplastic lesion, this issue is not resolved. FNH can also be associated with hereditary hemorrhagic telangiectasia (Osler-Weber-Rendu disease) or congenital absence of portal vein.[38–41] The characteristic features include a central scar with radiating fibrous bands, best visualized on trichrome and reticulin stains, forming incomplete, pseudocirrhotic nodules. The central scar contains thick-walled arteries. A marked ductular reaction and inflammatory

Fig. 2. (C) GS is absent within the tumor. Normal liver (*left*) shows pericentral cytoplasmic staining. (*D*) LFABP is negative within tumor (*left*), and faintly positive in normal liver (*right*).

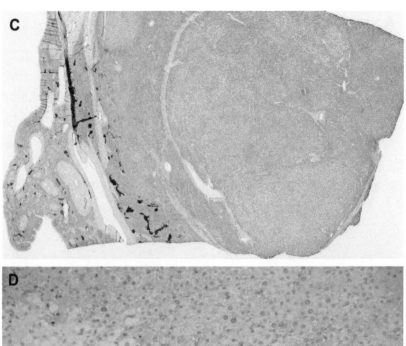

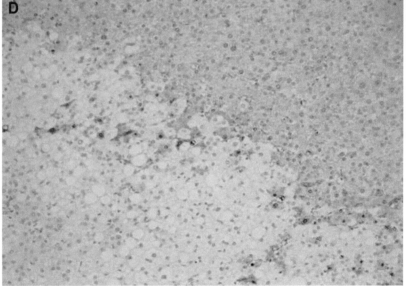

infiltrate are seen at the interface between the fibrous bands and hepatocytic nodules (**Fig. 5**). Although the diagnosis is straightforward in most resection specimens, its differentiation from HA and occasionally well-differentiated HCC can be challenging in core biopsies. It may mimic cirrhosis closely in some cases (hence, it was also called focal cirrhosis in the past); the clinical/imaging findings, and the background liver biopsy, if available, can help avoid this trap. IHC markers, including CK7, CK19, GS, SAA, CD34, and GPC3, can be helpful in difficult cases (**Table 3**). The entire panel of markers is not necessary and a limited panel can be used depending on the differential diagnosis in a given case. The proliferating immature ductules within the fibrous bands can be highlighted with CK7 and CK19 (**Fig. 5**), a feature usually absent in HA (except inflammatory subtype) and HCC. In FNH, GS characteristically stains large areas of hepatocytes around the central veins, in a "map-like", geographic pattern (**Fig. 5**),[42] and is the best marker for differentiating FNH from other hepatocellular nodules.[42,43]

HCC

The diagnosis of well-differentiated and moderately differentiated HCC and their differentiation from HA and FNH was discussed earlier.

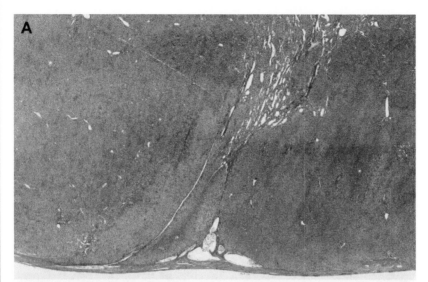

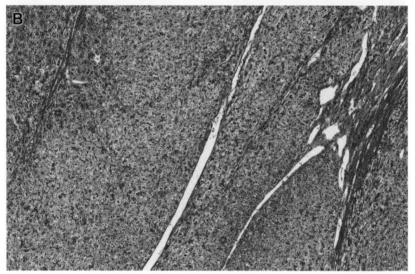

Fig. 3. β-catenin activated HA. (*A, B*) HA composed of 1-cell to 2-cell trabeculae, with mild significant cytologic atypia (hematoxylin-eosin, original magnification ×10, ×30).

POORLY DIFFERENTIATED TUMORS OF UNCLEAR LINEAGE

Tumors that are clearly malignant and are poorly differentiated require additional IHC markers to establish the cell of origin. Differential diagnosis includes HCC, CC, mixed HCC/CC, other primary liver tumors, and metastases. Clinical history and imaging are of the utmost importance before embarking on a shotgun approach with IHC stains. After clinical history and imaging are obtained, the first step should be to assess the basic morphologic pattern of the tumor based on hematoxylin-eosin stain and form a broad differential diagnosis. The markers that are often useful in

establishing the cell lineage as hepatocytic are discussed in detail later (Table 4).

Cholangiocarcinoma

CC represents 15% to 20% of all hepatic malignant epithelial neoplasms in the Western world, and are second only to HCC, which constitutes the remaining 80%. Most CC are easily recognized as gland-forming adenocarcinomas, and the major differential diagnosis is metastatic adenocarcinoma; however, some may have solid areas and may be difficult to differentiate from HCC and mixed tumors. The typical prominent desmoplastic stroma often helps to differentiate CC from

Fig. 3. (*C*) Diffuse cytoplasmic staining with GS within tumor cells. (*D*) Aberrant nuclear stain with β-catenin.

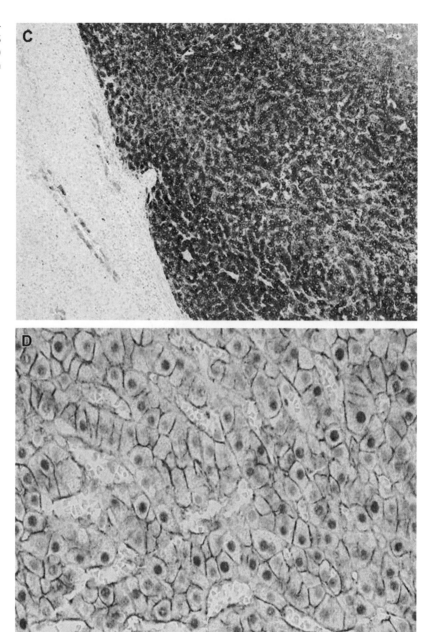

other metastatic adenocarcinomas; however, this is neither always present nor specific. CC is usually positive for CK7, CK19, CK8/18, may express CK20 and CDX2 in 40% cases, and is negative for the hepatocytic markers (HepPar-1 antigen, Arg1, and GPC3). pCEA stains the cytoplasm and membrane of tumor cells, unlike the canalicular pattern seen in HCC.[44] Villin, a restricted protein of the gastrointestinal tract, is expressed in approximately 50% of CCs, typically in a brush border pattern[45]; in contrast, hepatocellular carcinomas may express villin, albeit in a bile canalicular pattern. There is a single report that CD5 expression can be used to distinguish HCC from CC, reportedly positive in 85% of CC and absent in HCC. However, this marker is less useful in differentiating the latter from metastatic carcinomas, because carcinomas from other sites, like breast, colon, and pancreas are also positive.[46] There is no reliable marker to distinguish intrahepatic CC from metastatic adenocarcinoma originating in stomach, gallbladder, pancreas, or extrahepatic

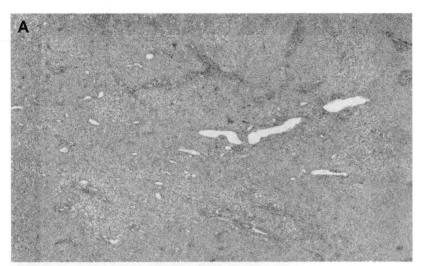

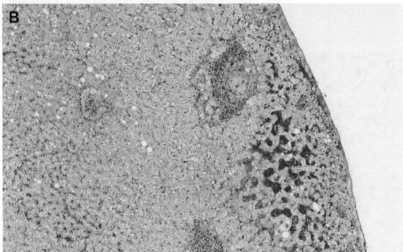

Fig. 4. Inflammatory HA. (*A*) HA, mild fatty infiltration, dilatation of arteries. and absent portal tracts (hematoxylin-eosin, original magnification ×10). (*B, C*) Marked sinusoidal dilatation and hemorrhage; perivascular inflammatory infiltrate, including lymphocytes, histiocytes, rare plasma cells. (*D*) Diffuse cytoplasmic staining with SAA.

bile ducts. Also, no IHC markers are available in distinguishing benign biliary proliferations from CC, and the diagnosis must be made on routine HE stains.

Mixed HCC-Cholangiocarcinoma

Mixed HCC-CC is less common; however, in our experience, it seems more common than the reported incidence of 1.0% to 3.5%.[47,48] These tumors contain unequivocal, intimately mixed elements of both HCC and CC. This tumor should be distinguished from separate HCC and CC arising in the same liver. The classic type contains areas of typical HCC and areas of typical CC; each type can be well-differentiated or moderately or poorly differentiated and is confirmed by mucin histochemistry and IHC staining with hepatocellular markers and CK7/CK19.[44] Cells that have phenotypical or immunophenotypical features of stem cells can be seen at the periphery of the tumor nodules, expressing CK7/CK19, CD56, C-kit, and epithelial cell adhesion molecule (EPCAM/MOC31); if these predominate, such tumors have been classified as combined HCC-CC with stem cell features.[12,49] The prognosis for combined HCC-CC without stem cell features is worse than HCC. The prognosis for combined HCC-CC with stem cell features is unknown, considering the small number of reported cases.[12]

Fig. 4.

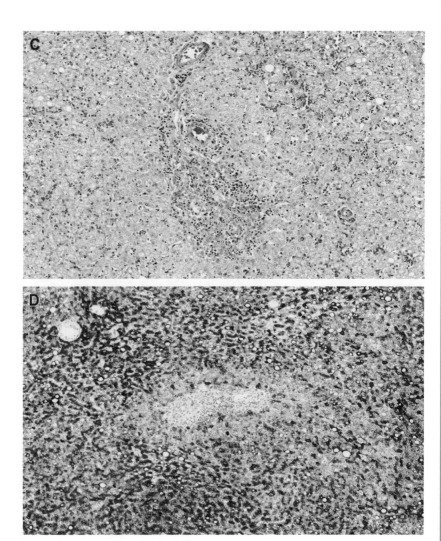

IHC MARKERS IN THE WORKUP OF HEPATOCYTIC LESIONS: USEFULNESS AND PITFALLS

Numerous IHC markers have been used in the work-up of hepatocytic lesions. A summary is provided in **Table 4**.

HepPar1

HepPar-1 is a monoclonal antibody that recognizes carbamyl phosphatase 1, an enzyme in the urea cycle. Immunoreactivity is typically seen as a diffuse cytoplasmic granular pattern. It is highly sensitive and specific for HCC, and is positive in most HCCs (75%–90%).[28]

Pitfalls in Diagnosis

HepPar-1 is negative in poorly differentiated and scirrhous-type HCC.[28] Staining can be patchy, and therefore unreliable in biopsies.[28,50] Although most adenocarcinomas are negative, HepPar-1 can be positive in gastric hepatoid carcinomas, esophageal, lung, pancreatic, urothelial, adrenocortical, colorectal, and uterine cervical carcinomas.[28,50,51]

ARG1

Arg1, an enzyme involved in the hydrolysis of arginine to ornithine and urea,[27] was recently recognized as a more sensitive and specific marker than HepPar-1, especially in poorly differentiated HCC.[27,52,53] It has diffuse cytoplasmic or nuclear

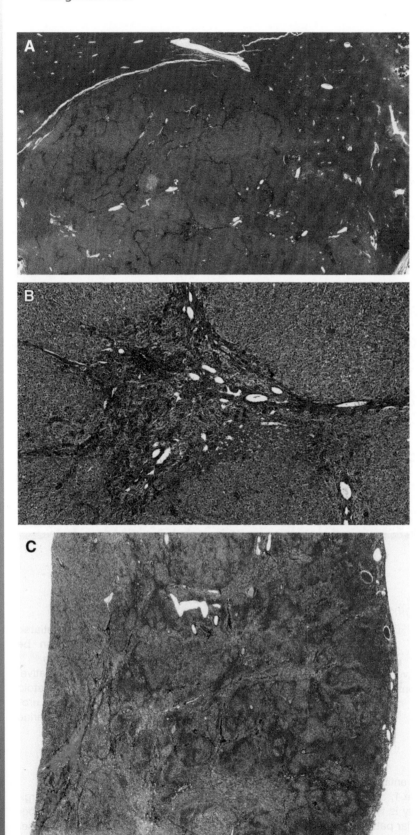

Fig. 5. FNH. (*A*) Well-circumscribed, multinodular lesion (hematoxylin-eosin, original magnification ×10). (*B*) The characteristic central scar with prominent blood vessels (hematoxylin-eosin, original magnification ×40), highlighted by Masson trichrome stain, along with the fibrous septa that give a pseudocirrhotic nodular appearance (*C*).

Fig. 5. (*D*) CK7 highlights bile ductular reaction around fibrous septa. (*E*) Characteristic "map-like" staining of FNH with GS. Normal liver stains a few hepatocytes around the central veins.

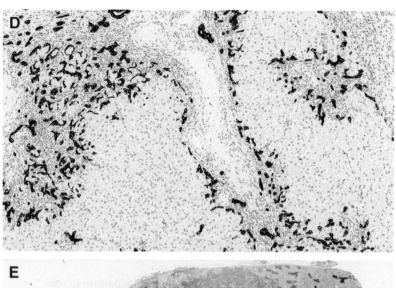

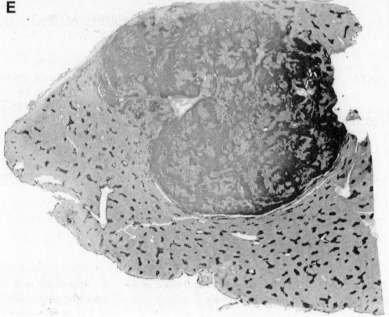

Table 4
IHC markers useful in the workup of hepatocytic lesions: usefulness and pitfalls

	Hepatocellular Carcinoma	
IHC Marker	Staining Pattern	Pitfalls
HepPar-1	Cytoplasmic, granular	Low sensitivity or absent in poorly differentiated and scirrhous HCC Patchy staining in biopsies Can be positive in gastric hepatoid, esophageal, lung, pancreatic, urothelial, adrenocortical, colorectal, and uterine cervical carcinomas
Arg1	Cytoplasmic and nuclear	May show minimal, patchy positivity in pancreatic carcinomas
GPC3	Cytoplasmic	Low sensitivity in well-differentiated HCC and in biopsies (<50%) Can be positive in melanoma, lung squamous carcinoma, germ cell tumors, and gastric hepatoid carcinomas Sometimes membranous or canalicular staining
GS	Cytoplasmic	Diffusely positive in β-catenin–activated HA-focal expression in HGDN Typical maplike pattern in FNH
α Fetoprotein	Cytoplasmic	Low sensitivity (25%–50%) Patchy staining Positive also in germ cell tumors
pCEA	Canalicular	Distinction between cytoplasmic staining in adenocarcinoma and canalicular pattern in HCC can be difficult Sensitivity in poorly differentiated HCC is low (25%–50%)
CD10	Canalicular	Low sensitivity (<50%) Does not differentiate between benign and malignant hepatocytic lesions Can show a membranous pattern staining
CD34	Sinusoidal	Can show incomplete staining in HGDN, HA, and FNH
Heat shock protein 70	Cytoplasmic and nuclear	Patchy staining in HCC

staining. Overall sensitivities of Arg1 and HepPar-1 are 96.0% and 84.1%, respectively.[53]

Pitfalls in Diagnosis

Arg1 staining may be seen also in some pancreatic adenocarcinomas, for which the liver is a frequent site of metastasis, however this was reported in a single study with very few cases that show high background staining.[27] Arg1, like HepPar-1, is positive in both normal and neoplastic liver, and has no role in the differentiation of well-differentiated HCC from HA or FNH.[27]

GLYPICAN 3

GPC3 is a member of the glypican family, a group of heparin sulfate proteoglycans linked to the cell surface through a glycosylphosphatidylinositol anchor that is expressed in fetal liver and placenta but not in adult liver.[28] Glypicans play an important role in cell growth, differentiation, and migration. GPC3 is highly expressed, both at the messenger RNA (mRNA) and protein level, in HCC.[26] Reactivation of the fetal phenotype, which is common in malignant tumors, may explain the expression of GPC3 in malignant hepatocellular nodules. GPC3 is expressed in 64% to 90% of HCC and is absent in HA, FNH, cirrhosis, and normal liver. However, the sensitivity of GPC3 in well-differentiated HCC is 50% and may be lower in needle biopsies.[50] GPC3 has a higher sensitivity than HepPar-1 in poorly differentiated HCC.[26,28,54,55]

Pitfalls in Diagnosis

GPC3 can be negative in well-differentiated HCC and the staining can be patchy. GPC3 is also positive in other tumors, including melanoma, squamous carcinoma of lung, germ cell tumors (yolk sac tumors and choriocarcinoma), and gastric hepatoid carcinomas.[26,28,54–56]

CARCINOEMBRYONIC ANTIGEN

Carcinoembryonic antigen (BGP) (CEA) is a family of proteins that includes true CEA, nonspecific cross-reacting antigen, and biliary glycoprotein (BGP). Using polyclonal antibodies to CEA which cross-react with both true CEA as well as BGP, a typical canalicular pattern is seen in 60% to 90% of well-differentiated to moderately differentiated HCC.[28,57,58] The staining reflects expression of BGP and not true CEA, and is not seen with monoclonal antibodies. Diffuse cytoplasmic expression of CEA is seen in most adenocarcinomas.[28,58]

Pitfalls in Diagnosis

BGP/CEA has a low sensitivity in poorly differentiated HCC (25%–50%). In addition to canalicular pattern, about half of HCC also show cytoplasmic staining.[28] In poorly differentiated HCC, there may not be distinct canalicular staining. Intense canalicular staining in HCC may mimic a membranous pattern of immunoreactivity, whereas weak or luminal staining in metastatic adenocarcinoma or CC may be misinterpreted as a canalicular pattern.[57] Sensitivity in poorly differentiated HCC is low (25%–50%).[28]

CD10

CD10[59] shows a canalicular staining pattern, similar to BGP, which is not seen in adenocarcinoma.[57]

Pitfalls in Diagnosis

CD10 does not differentiate between benign and malignant hepatocytic lesions.[59] It can also show a membranous pattern staining. It has a low sensitivity (50%) and is not specific for HCC, making it a less useful antibody.[60]

CYTOKERATINS

Normal and neoplastic hepatocytes express CK8/18 and are negative for CK 7, CK19, and CK20.[28,61] Therefore, most HCC stain with antibodies to low-molecular-weight keratin (eg, CAM5.2), but not with antibodies to high-molecular-weight cytokeratin (eg, 34βE12).[62] Keratin AE1/AE3 is a mixture of AE1 and AE3 clones, of which AE1 reacts with type I keratins (CK10, CK15–16, and CK19) and AE3 reacts with type II keratins (CK1–6 and CK8).[63] A well-balanced AE1/AE3 cocktail cannot be used to separate hepatocellular carcinoma from adenocarcinoma.

α FETOPROTEIN

α Fetoprotein (AFP) is an oncofetal protein produced by the liver and visceral endoderm of the yolk sac. It is expressed in neoplastic hepatic tissues but not in normal liver; other tumors only rarely express AFP (germ cell tumors).

Pitfalls in Diagnosis

Only about 25% to 40% of cases of HCC are positive for AFP by IHC and the staining tends to be patchy.[28,58,60,64] Serum AFP levels are more often increased with HCC, and more helpful in establishing the diagnosis and monitoring response to therapy for HCC.

HEAT SHOCK PROTEIN 70

Heat shock protein 70 (HSP70) is an antiapoptotic gene that was found through mRNA expression profiling to be upregulated in HCC, but not in the adjacent normal liver. HSPs, the so-called stress proteins, are a large group of highly conserved proteins that are expressed by prokaryotes and eukaryotes. The HSPs are a family of molecular chaperones, which share the properties of modifying protein structures and interactions between target proteins and other proteins. HSPs can be classified by molecular weight, and include HSP15 to HSP30, HSP40, HSP60, HSP70, HSP90, and HSP100. HSP70 is of special relevance in human cancer because it inhibits cancer cell apoptosis.[65] A strong association between tumor size, vascular invasion, histologic grade, and HSP70 overexpression has been reported.[65]

HSP70 is overexpressed by IHC (nuclear and cytoplasmic staining) and reverse transcriptase polymerase chain reaction in early HCC compared with preneoplastic lesions and in progressed HCC compared with early HCC.[66] HSP70 is expressed by IHC in 80% of HCC in resection specimens, but less than 50% in biopsies.[50,67,68] In our experience, the positivity in HCC is even less frequent. Bile duct epithelium shows cytoplasmic staining for HSP70, and therefore can be used as an internal control.

When 3 antibodies were used (GPC3, HSP70, and GS), the specificity and sensitivity for diagnosis of HCC was 100% and 57%, respectively, when 2 of the 3 antibodies were expressed.[50,67–69]

With CD34, neovascularization is an important biological process for tumor growth and metastasis. For most tumors, this process usually occurs in the stroma adjacent to the tumor. In HCC, neo-vascularization is unique because direct capillarization occurs in sinusoidal spaces in tumor tissue.[54] CD34 antibody strongly stains the endothelial lining cells of HCC, in contrast to the minimal reactivity of sinusoidal endothelial cells confined to the vicinity of portal tracts in normal liver and in the periphery of cirrhotic nodules. This staining is attributed to a capillarization of sinusoids, leading to a change in the phenotype of endothelial cells.[12,28,70,71] This pattern is not seen in adenocarcinomas.[28] In some situations, CD34 can be useful in the distinction of a well-differentiated necrotic neoplasm from cirrhotic or normal liver in small biopsies.[28,54] CD34 staining is one of the important markers of tumor angiogenesis and microvascular density in HCC and is closely associated with HCC prognosis.[72]

Pitfalls in Diagnosis

Although the specificity is high for HCC, the sensitivity is low (20%–40%). CD34 can show occasionally diffuse staining in HA and FNH.[28,54]

GLUTAMINE SYNTHETASE

GS is an enzyme that combines glutamate with ammonia to produce glutamine, and its most important function is to aid in ammonia detoxification. The GS gene is upregulated as a result of nuclear translocation of β-catenin. In normal liver, GS is expressed only by 1 or 2 layers of hepatocytes around the central veins.[21,31] GS is diffusely positive (cytoplasmic) in HCC (50%–70%)[65,73] but also in β-catenin–activated HA.[31,50] The other subtypes of HA are negative, or show weak and patchy positivity, or rarely pseudomaplike positivity.[50] In FNH, GS has a typical, maplike pattern.[35,42]

MOC31 (EPCAM)

MOC31 (EPCAM) is an antibody against a cell surface glycoprotein and was initially used to separate mesothelioma from metastatic adenocarcinoma.[28,74] In liver biopsies, it consistently shows membranous staining in most metastatic adenocarcinomas and CCs, although staining in HCC is negative or weakly, patchy positive.[28,75,76]

The most useful ancillary tools in the setting of well-differentiated hepatocellular neoplasms in noncirrhotic liver are GPC3, β-catenin, and GS. Expression of GPC3, nuclear staining with β-catenin, and diffuse cytoplasmic staining with GS strongly favor well-differentiated HCC. In the setting of poorly differentiated HCC, useful IHC markers include GPC3, Arg1, GS, and MOC31.

METASTATIC CARCINOMAS

Once the hepatocytic lineage has been excluded from the differential diagnosis based on clinical history, tumor morphology, or special stains, metastases and other rare primary tumors need to be excluded. The first and foremost goal should be to obtain a good clinical history of any previous known malignancy, and sometimes a telephone call to the primary care physician goes a long way in saving unnecessary and extensive workup. If there is a known history of previous malignancy, comparison with the previous histology is a good idea. The next step should be to look at the histologic features carefully and recognize if the tumor can be classified in any of the 5 well-defined histologic patterns outlined as follows:

1. Tumors composed of large polygonal cells arranged in trabecular, nested, compact, or solid architecture: the differential diagnosis includes metastatic carcinomas, HCC, poorly differentiated CC, epithelioid AML metastatic melanoma, endocrine tumors, and sarcomas with epithelioid morphology (**Fig. 6**).
2. Tumors with obvious glandular/acinar/papillary differentiation: these include metastatic adenocarcinomas from various sites and need to be differentiated from CC (**Fig. 7**). This distinction may not be always possible based on morphology and immunohistochemistry.
3. Tumors with squamous differentiation: these include metastatic squamous cell carcinoma of various sites, or tumors with prominent squamous component like endometrioid adenocarcinoma or mucoepidermoid tumor (**Fig. 8A–F**).
4. Tumors with clear cells: these include metastatic renal cell carcinoma, adrenal cortical carcinoma, and melanoma. These tumors need to be differentiated from the clear cell variant of HCC and CC with clear cells (**Fig. 9**).
5. Tumors with organoid (neuroendocrine) architecture (either small or large cells): these include metastatic neuroendocrine neoplasms, usually of pancreatic or pulmonary origin, but can come from any other sites, including gastrointestinal tract, prostate, or genital tract (**Fig. 8G, I**).

Based on the morphologic pattern, the IHC markers required can be narrowed down to the most useful panel depending on the primary site (**Table 5**). The most common of these patterns encountered in clinical practice is the glandular

Fig. 6. Liver tumors of uncertain lineage showing solid pattern. (*A*) HCC, solid pattern. The tumor is diffusely positive for HepPar-1 (*B*) Metastatic malignant melanoma (*C*), forming solid sheets of highly pleomorphic cells with numerous atypical mitoses. Another example showing strong reactivity with Melan A (*D*).

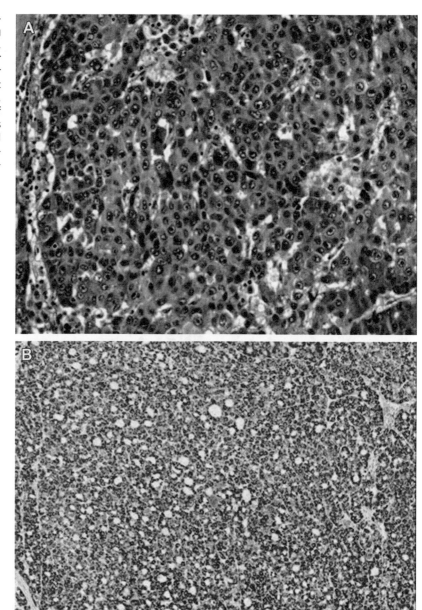

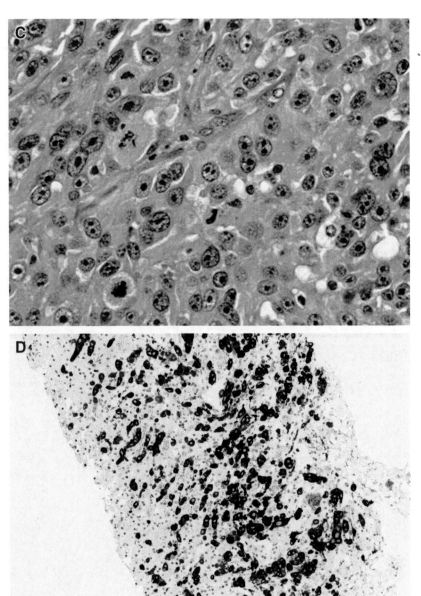

Fig. 6.

Fig. 7. Metastatic tumors in liver, glandular pattern. (*A*) Typical glandular formation in a desmoplastic stroma with focal mucin production. The tumor expresses nuclear ER (*B*) and cytoplasmic mammaglobin (*C*), consistent with breast origin.

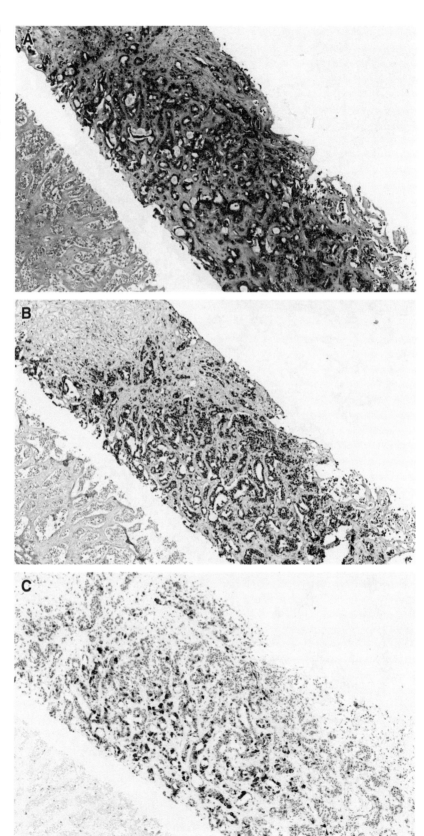

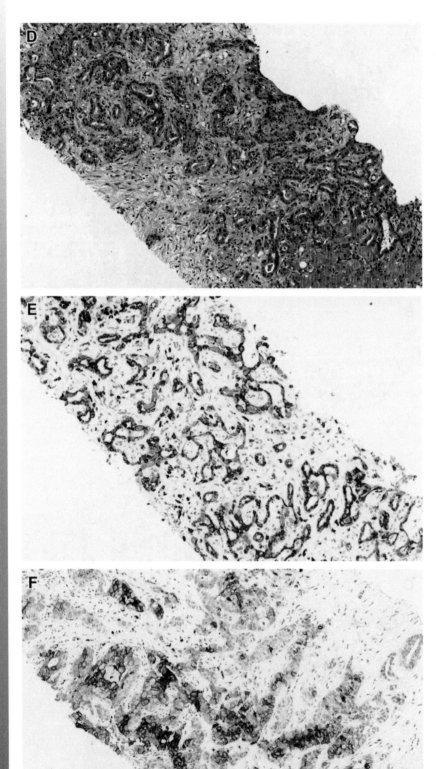

Fig. 7. (*D*) CC with dense desmoplastic stroma. Positive cytoplasmic immunoreactive CD5 (*E*), positive cytoplasmic pCEA (*F*). The tumor also expressed CK7, MUC1, and no expression of TTF1 and HepPar-1 (not shown).

Fig. 7. (G) Metastatic lung adenocarcinoma. The tumor cells show strong nuclear thyroid transcription factor 1 (*H*) and cytoplasmic staining with CK7 (*I*). No expression was seen with CK20 and CD5 (not shown).

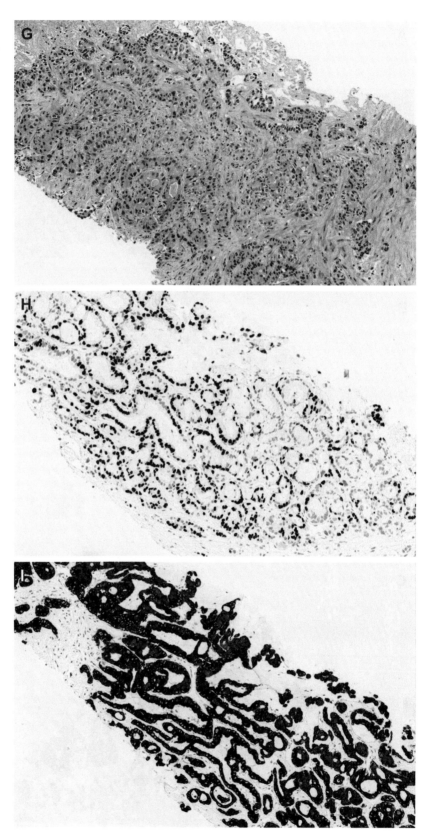

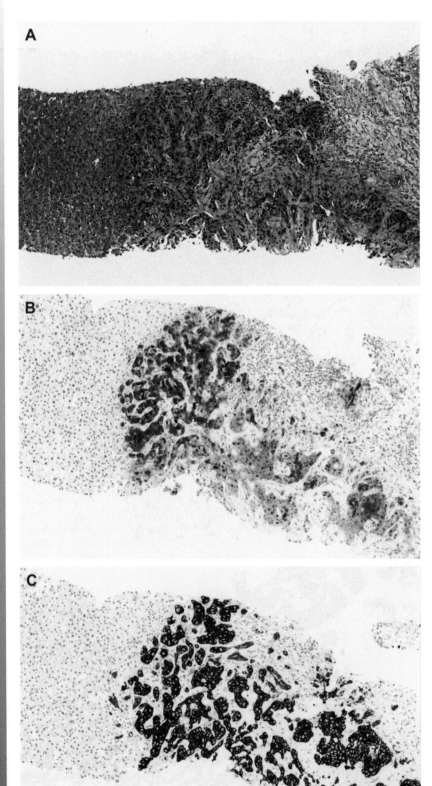

Fig. 8. Metastatic tumors with squamous differentiation. (*A*) Metastatic vulvar adenosquamous carcinoma. The tumor show strong expression with p16 (*B*) and CK7 (*C*). No expression was seen with HepPar-1, CEAp, MUC2, MUC5AC, TTF1, PAX8, CK5, p63, and CDX2 (not shown).

Fig. 8. (D) Metastatic squamous cell carcinoma originating from a soft palate tumor. The tumor is strongly positive for CK5 (*E*) and p63 (*F*).

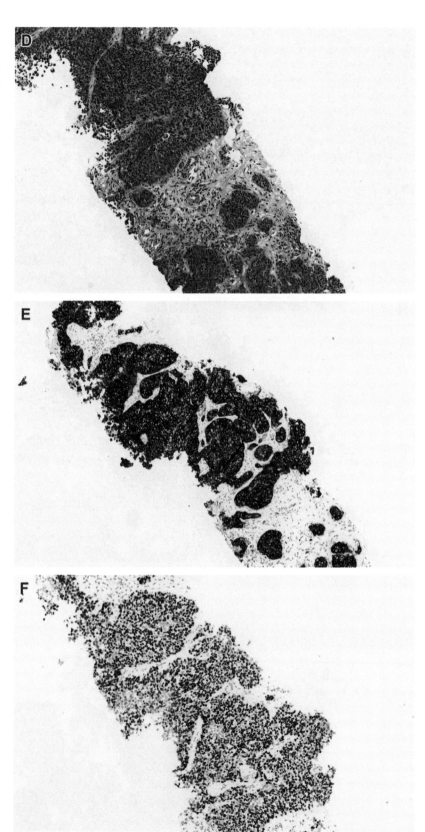

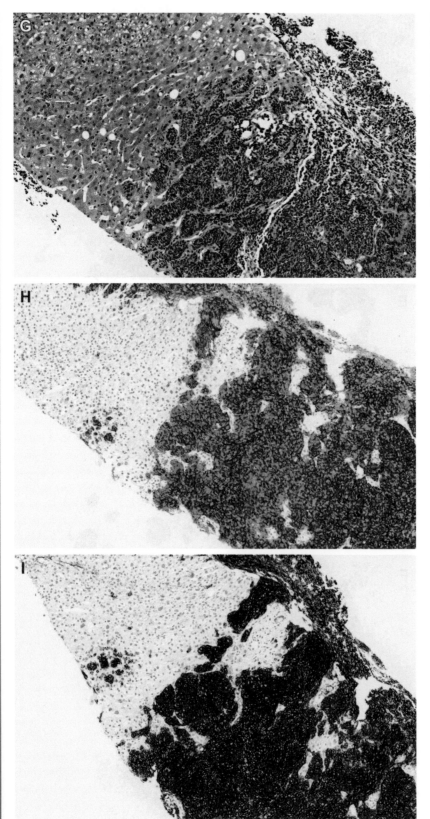

Fig. 8. (*G*) Metastatic carcinomas with organoid architecture. Metastatic small cell carcinoma of lung origin (*G*). Tumnor cells show scant cytoplasm, hyperchromatic, small nuclei, and prominent nuclear molding. The tumor expressed strong reactivity with synaptophysin (*H*) and CD56 (*I*), as well as thyroid transcription factor (not shown).

Fig. 9. Malignant tumors with clear cytoplasm. (*A*) HCC with clear cells. The tumor shows a trabecular pattern, and cells have centrally placed nuclei and abundant clear cytoplasm. Tumor cells expressed cytoplasmic AFP (*B*) and HepPar-1 (not shown).

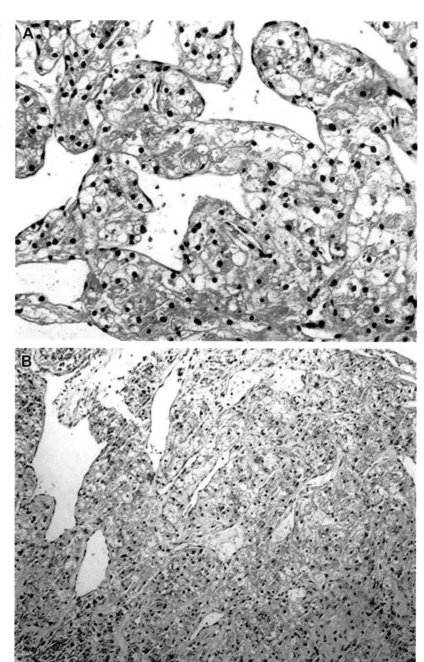

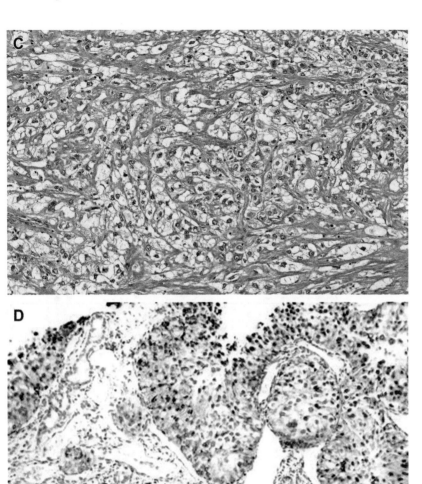

Fig. 9. (C) Metastatic renal cell carcinoma, clear cell type. Tumor cells expressed RCC (D) as well as EMA and vimentin (not shown).

Fig. 9. (*E*) Metastatic pancreatic carcinoma with clear cells. Tumor cells expressed CK7 (*F*).

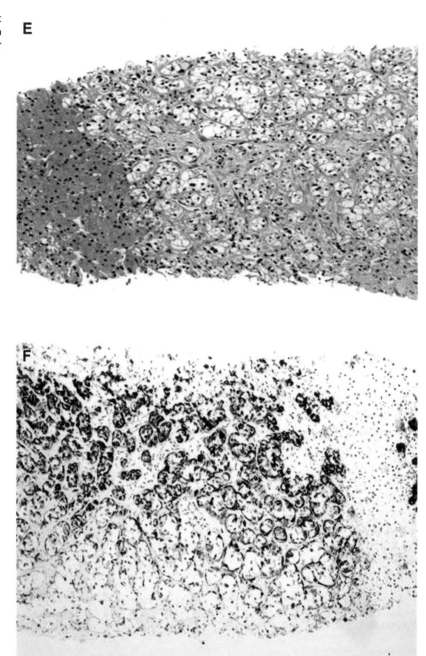

Table 5
Most commonly used IHC stains in the differential diagnosis of hepatic metastatic carcinomas of unknown primary and tumors of unclear lineage

Tumor Type	MOC31	HepPar-1, GPC3, or Arg1	Pertinent Positive Markers
HCC	−	+	pCEA[a], CD34[b], CD10[a], villin[a], GS, AFP
CC	+	−	CK7, CK19, CD5, CK 8/18, CK20 (40%), pCEA (cytoplasmic), CDX2
Colorectal adenocarcinoma	+	−	CK20, CDX2, villin, MUC2
Pancreatic adenocarcinoma	+	−	CK8/18, CK17, CK19, CK7, IMP3, MUC1, MUC4, MUC5AC, MUC2 (intestinal type), CA19-9
Lung adenocarcinoma	+	−	CK7, TTF1, napsin A, surfactant A, MUC1
Squamous cell carcinoma	+	−	p63, p40, CK5/6
Neuroendocrine tumors	+	−	CD56, synaptophysin, chromogranin, TTF1, AE1/3
Endometrium carcinoma	+	−	CK7, ER, PR, β-catenin, vimentin, Pax8, CA125, CD138
Ovarian serous	+	−	CK7, Pax8, CA125, ER, PR, WT1, mesothelin, vimentin, MUC1
Ovarian mucinous carcinoma	+	−	CK7, CK20, Pax8, CDX2, mCEA, E-cadherin
Prostate adenocarcinoma	+	−	AMACR (not specific for prostate), PSA, PAP, AE1/3, NKX3.1, ERG (Ets-related gene)
Renal clear cell carcinoma	+	−	RCC, vimentin, EMA, CD10, Pax8, Pax2
Renal chromophobe carcinoma	+	−	CD117, CK7, E-cadherin, Pax8, EMA
Renal papillary carcinoma	+	−	CK7, RCC, Pax8, AMACR, Pax2, RCC, EMA
Malignant Melanoma	−	−	S100, HMB45, Melan A, MART1, tyrosinase
Adrenal gland carcinoma	−	−	AE1/3, Melan A, calretinin, inhibin, CD56
Testicular seminomatous tumors	±	−	CD117, OCT3/4, PLAP, SALL4
Testicular nonseminomatous (germ cell tumors)	±	−	AE1/3, CD30, CK8/18/CAM5.2, CD10, PLAP (60%), HCG, SALL4
Bladder transitional carcinoma	+	−	CK7, CK20, CK5, p63, GATA3, E-cadherin, uroplakin III
Vascular tumors	−	−	CD31, CD34, FLI-1, ERG
AML	−	−	HMB45, Melan A, MART1, actin HHF-35, CD68, TFE3 (transcription factor E3)[77]

[a] Canalicular.
[b] Sinusoidal.

pattern. This is certainly not an all-inclusive list and virtually any tumor can metastasize to the liver, and needs to be considered in the context of appropriate histology, immunophenotype, clinical history, and serum tumor markers.

REFERENCES

1. International Consensus Group for Hepatocellular Neoplasia. Pathologic diagnosis of early hepatocellular carcinoma: a report of the international consensus group for hepatocellular neoplasia. Hepatology 2009;49(2):658–64.
2. Park YN. Update on precursor and early lesions of hepatocellular carcinomas. Arch Pathol Lab Med 2011;135(6):704–15.
3. Park YN, Yang CP, Fernandez GJ, et al. Neoangiogenesis and sinusoidal "capillarization" in dysplastic nodules of the liver. Am J Surg Pathol 1998;22(6): 656–62.
4. Park YN, Kojiro M, Di Tommaso L, et al. Ductular reaction is helpful in defining early stromal invasion,

small hepatocellular carcinomas, and dysplastic nodules. Cancer 2007;109(5):915–23.

5. Roncalli M, Terracciano L, Di Tommaso L, et al. Liver precancerous lesions and hepatocellular carcinoma: the histology report. Dig Liver Dis 2011;43: S361–72.

6. Kojiro M, Nakashima O. Histopathologic evaluation of hepatocellular carcinoma with special reference to small early stage tumors. Semin Liver Dis 1999; 19(3):287–96.

7. Bruix J, Sherman M. Management of hepatocellular carcinoma. Hepatology 2005;42(5):1208–36.

8. de Lope CR, Tremosini S, Forner A, et al. Management of HCC. J Hepatol 2012;56:S75–87.

9. Forner A, Vilana R, Ayuso C, et al. Diagnosis of hepatic nodules 20 mm or smaller in cirrhosis: prospective validation of the noninvasive diagnostic criteria for hepatocellular carcinoma. Hepatology 2008;47(1):97–104.

10. Sherman M. Hepatocellular carcinoma: epidemiology, surveillance, and diagnosis. Semin Liver Dis 2010;30(1):3–16.

11. Bruix J, Sherman M. Management of hepatocellular carcinoma: an update. Hepatology 2011;53(3): 1020–2.

12. Mitchell KA, Jain D. Diagnostic approach to needle biopsies of hepatic mass lesions. Diagn Histopathol 2008;14(12):598–608.

13. Quaglia A, Tibballs J, Grasso A. Focal nodular hyperplasia-like areas in cirrhosis. Histopathology 2003;42(1):14–21.

14. Nakashima O, Kurogi M, Yamaguchi R. Unique hypervascular nodules in alcoholic liver cirrhosis: identical to focal nodular hyperplasia-like nodules? J Hepatol 2004;41(6):992–8.

15. Sasaki M, Yoneda N, Kitamura S. A serum amyloid A-positive hepatocellular neoplasm arising in alcoholic cirrhosis: a previously unrecognized type of inflammatory hepatocellular tumor. Mod Pathol 2012;25(12):1584–93.

16. Torbenson M. Review of the clinicopathologic features of fibrolamellar carcinoma. Adv Anat Pathol 2007;14(3):217–23.

17. Klein WM, Molmenti EP, Colombani PM, et al. Primary liver carcinoma arising in people younger than 30 years. Am J Clin Pathol 2005;124(4):512–8.

18. Ross HM, Daniel HD, Vivekanandan P, et al. Fibrolamellar carcinomas are positive for CD68. Mod Pathol 2011;24(3):390–5.

19. Bioulac-Sage P, Cubel G, Balabaud C. Pathological diagnosis of hepatocellular adenoma in clinical practice. Diagn Histopathol 2011;17(12): 521–9.

20. Reznik Y, Dao T, Coutant R, et al. Hepatocyte nuclear factor-1 alpha gene inactivation: cosegregation between liver. J Clin Endocrinol Metab 2004; 89(3):1476–80.

21. Bioulac-Sage P, Balabaud C, Zucman-Rossi J. Subtype classification of hepatocellular adenoma. Dig Surg 2010;27:39–45.

22. Bioulac-Sage P, Laumonier H, Laurent C, et al. Hepatocellular adenoma: what is new in 2008. Hepatol Int 2008;2(3):316–21.

23. Rebouissou S, Bioulac-Sage P, Zucman-Rossi J. Molecular pathogenesis of focal nodular hyperplasia and hepatocellular adenoma. J Hepatol 2008; 48:163–70.

24. Foster JH, Berman MM. The malignant transformation of liver cell adenomas. Arch Surg 1994;129(7): 712–7.

25. Yamauchi N, Watanabe A, Hishinuma M, et al. The glypican 3 oncofetal protein is a promising diagnostic marker for hepatocellular carcinoma. Mod Pathol 2005;18(12):1591–8.

26. Wang XY, Degos F, Dubois S, et al. Glypican-3 expression in hepatocellular tumors: diagnostic value for preneoplastic lesions and hepatocellular carcinomas. Hum Pathol 2006;37:1435–41.

27. Fujiwara M, Kwok S, Yano H, et al. Arginase-1 is a more sensitive marker of hepatic differentiation than HepPar-1 and glypican-3 in fine-needle aspiration biopsies. Cancer Cytopathol 2012;120(4): 230–7.

28. Kakar S, Gown AM, Goodman ZD, et al. Best practices in diagnostic immunohistochemistry: hepatocellular carcinoma versus metastatic neoplasms. Arch Pathol Lab Med 2007;131:1648–54.

29. Kong CS, Appenzeller M, Ferrell LD. Utility of CD34 reactivity in evaluating focal nodular hepatocellular lesions sampled by fine needle aspiration biopsy. Acta Cytol 2000;44(2):218–22.

30. Bioulac-Sage P, Laumonier H, Couchy G, et al. Hepatocellular adenoma management and phenotypic classification: the Bordeaux experience. Hepatology 2009;50(2):481–9.

31. Bioulac-Sage P, Rebouissou S, Thomas C, et al. Hepatocellular adenoma subtype classification using molecular markers and immunohistochemistry. Hepatology 2007;46(3):740–8.

32. Bellanné-Chantelot C, Carette C, Riveline J-P, et al. The type and the position of HNF1A mutation modulate age at diagnosis of diabetes in patients with maturity-onset diabetes of the young (MODY)-3. Diabetes 2008;57(2):503–8.

33. Bioulac-Sage P, Balabaud C, Bedossa P, et al. Pathological diagnosis of liver cell adenoma and focal nodular hyperplasia: Bordeaux update. J Hepatol 2007;46:521–7.

34. Bacq Y, Jacquemin E, Balabaud C, et al. Familial liver adenomatosis associated with hepatocyte nuclear factor 1alpha inactivation. Gastroenterology 2003;125:1470–5.

35. Bioulac-Sage P, Laumonier H, Balabaud C. Benign hepatocellular tumors. In: Saxena R, editor.

Practical hepatic pathology, 34. Philadelphia: Saunders; 2010. p. 473–88.

36. Bioulac-Sage P, Cubel G, Balabaud C, et al. Revisiting the pathology of resected benign hepatocellular nodules using new immunohistochemical markers. Semin Liver Dis 2011;31(1):91–103.

37. Bioulac-Sage P, Rebouissou S, Sa Cunha A, et al. Clinical, morphologic, and molecular features defining so-called telangiectatic focal nodular hyperplasias of the liver. Gastroenterology 2005;128:1211–8.

38. Bioulac-Sage P, Balabaud C, Zucman-Rossi J. Focal nodular hyperplasia, hepatocellular adenomas: past, present, future. Gastroenterol Clin Biol 2010;34:355–8.

39. Altavilla G, Guariso G. Focal nodular hyperplasia of the liver associated with portal vein agenesis: a morphological and immunohistochemical study of one case and review of the literature. Adv Clin Path 1999;3(4):139–45.

40. Buscarini E, Danesino C, Plauchu H, et al. High prevalence of hepatic focal nodular hyperplasia in subjects with hereditary hemorrhagic telangiectasia. Ultrasound Med Biol 2004;30: 1089–97.

41. De Gaetano AM, Gui B, Macis G, et al. Congenital absence of the portal vein associated with focal nodular hyperplasia in the liver in an adult woman: imaging and review of the literature. Abdom Imaging 2004;29(4):455–9.

42. Bioulac-Sage P, Laumonier H, Rullier A, et al. Overexpression of glutamine synthetase in focal nodular hyperplasia: a novel easy diagnostic tool in surgical pathology. Liver Int 2009;29(3):459–65.

43. Tsai JH, Jeng YM, Pan CC, et al. Immunostaining of glutamine synthetase is a sensitive and specific marker for diagnosing focal nodular hyperplasia in needle biopsy. Pathology 2012;44(7):605–10.

44. Ryu HS, Lee K, Shin E, et al. Comparative analysis of immunohistochemical markers for differential diagnosis of hepatocelluar carcinoma and cholangiocarcinoma. Tumori 2012;98(4):478–84.

45. Werling RW, Yaziji H, Bacchi CE, et al. CDX2, a highly sensitive and specific marker of adenocarcinomas of intestinal origin: an immunohistochemical survey of 476 primary and metastatic carcinomas. Am J Surg Pathol 2003;27(3):303–10.

46. Chu PG, Arber DA, Weiss LM. Expression of T/NK-cell and plasma cell antigens in nonhematopoietic epithelioid neoplasms. An immunohistochemical study of 447 cases. Am J Clin Pathol 2003;120(1): 64–70.

47. Fukukura Y, Taguchi J, Nakashima O, et al. Combined hepatocellular and cholangiocarcinoma: correlation between CT findings. J Comput Assist Tomogr 1997;21(1):52–8.

48. Yano Y, Yamamoto J, Kosuge T, et al. Combined hepatocellular and cholangiocarcinoma: a clinicopathologic study of 26. Jpn J Clin Oncol 2003;33(6):283–7.

49. Zhang F, Chen XP, Zhang W, et al. Combined hepatocellular cholangiocarcinoma originating from hepatic progenitor cells: immunohistochemical and double-fluorescence immunostaining evidence. Histopathology 2008;52(2):224–32.

50. Shafizadeh N, Kakar S. Diagnosis of well-differentiated hepatocellular lesions: role of immunohistochemistry and other ancillary techniques. Adv Anat Pathol 2011;18:438–45.

51. Krishna M. Diagnosis of metastatic neoplasms: an immunohistochemical approach. Arch Pathol Lab Med 2010;134:207–15.

52. Timek DT, Shi J, Liu H, et al. Arginase-1, HepPar-1, and Glypican-3 are the most effective panel of markers in distinguishing hepatocellular carcinoma from metastatic tumor on fine-needle aspiration specimens. Am J Clin Pathol 2012;138:203–10.

53. Yan BC, Gong C, Song J, et al. Arginase-1: a new immunohistochemical marker of hepatocytes and hepatocellular neoplasms. Am J Surg Pathol 2010;34:1147–54.

54. Coston WM, Loera S, Lau SK, et al. Distinction of hepatocellular carcinoma from benign hepatic mimickers using Glypican-3 and CD34 immunohistochemistry. Am J Surg Pathol 2008;32(3): 433–44.

55. Wang FH, Yip YC, Zhang M, et al. Diagnostic utility of glypican-3 for hepatocellular carcinoma on liver needle biopsy. J Clin Pathol 2010;63: 599–603.

56. Hishinuma M, Ohashi KI, Yamauchi N, et al. Hepatocellular oncofetal protein, glypican 3 is a sensitive marker for alpha-fetoprotein-producing gastric carcinoma. Histopathology 2006;49:479–86.

57. Morrison C, Marsh W Jr, Frankel WL. A comparison of CD10 to pCEA, MOC-31, and hepatocyte for the distinction of malignant tumors in the liver. Mod Pathol 2002;15(12):1279–87.

58. Lau SK, Prakash S, Geller SA, et al. Comparative immunohistochemical profile of hepatocellular carcinoma, cholangiocarcinoma, and metastatic adenocarcinoma. Hum Pathol 2002;33:1175–81.

59. Borscheri N, Roessner A, Rocken C. Canalicular immunostaining of neprilysin (CD10) as a diagnostic marker for hepatocellular carcinomas. Am J Surg Pathol 2001;25(10):1297–303.

60. Wang L, Vuolo M, Suhrland MJ, et al. HepPar1, MOC-31, pCEA, mCEA and CD10 for distinguishing hepatocellular carcinoma vs. metastatic adenocarcinoma in liver fine needle aspirates. Acta Cytol 2006;50(3):257–62.

61. Maeda T, Kajiyama K, Adachi E. The expression of cytokeratins 7, 19, and 20 in primary and metastatic carcinomas of the liver. Mod Pathol 1996;9(9): 901–9.

62. Gown AM, Vogel AM. Monoclonal antibodies to human intermediate filament proteins. III. Analysis of tumors. Am J Clin Pathol 1985;84(4):413–24.

63. Oien KA. Pathologic evaluation of unknown primary cancer. Semin Oncol 2009;36:8–37.

64. Chu PG, Ishizawa S, Wu E, et al. Hepatocyte antigen as a marker of hepatocellular carcinoma: an immunohistochemical comparison to carcinoembryonic antigen, CD10, and alpha-fetoprotein. Am J Surg Pathol 2002;26(8):978–88.

65. Shin E, Ryu HS, Kim SH, et al. The clinicopathological significance of heat shock protein 70 and glutamine synthetase expression in hepatocellular carcinoma. J Hepatobiliary Pancreat Sci 2011;18(4):544–50.

66. Chuma M, Sakamoto M, Yamazaki K, et al. Expression profiling in multistage hepatocarcinogenesis: identification of HSP70. Hepatology 2003;37(1):198–207.

67. Di Tommaso L, Destro A, Seok JY, et al. The application of markers (HSP70 GPC3 and GS) in liver biopsies is useful for detection of hepatocellular carcinoma. J Hepatol 2009;50(4):746–54.

68. Di Tommaso L, Franchi G, Park YN, et al. Diagnostic value of HSP70, glypican 3, and glutamine synthetase in hepatocellular nodules in cirrhosis. Hepatology 2007;45(3):725–34.

69. Tremosini S, Forner A, Boix L, et al. Prospective validation of an immunohistochemical panel (glypican 3, heat shock protein 70 and glutamine synthetase) in liver biopsies for diagnosis of very early hepatocellular carcinoma. Gut 2012;61:1481–7.

70. Ahmad I, Iyer A, Marginean CE, et al. Diagnostic use of cytokeratins, CD34, and neuronal cell adhesion molecule staining in focal nodular hyperplasia and hepatic adenoma. Hum Pathol 2009;40(5):726–34.

71. Ruck P, Xiao JC, Kaiserling E. Immunoreactivity of sinusoids in hepatocellular carcinoma. An immunohistochemical study using lectin UEA-1 and antibodies against endothelial markers, including CD34. Arch Pathol Lab Med 1995;119(2):173–8.

72. Wang F, Jing X, Wang T, et al. Differential diagnostic value of GPC3-CD34 combined staining in small liver nodules with diameter less than 3 cm. Am J Clin Pathol 2012;137(6):937–45.

73. Long J, Wang H, Lang Z. Expression level of glutamine synthetase is increased in hepatocellular carcinoma. Hepatol Int 2011;5(2):698–706.

74. Ordonez NG. Value of the MOC-31 monoclonal antibody in differentiating epithelial pleural mesothelioma from lung adenocarcinoma. Hum Pathol 1998;29:166–9.

75. Niemann TH, Hughes JH, De Young BR. MOC-31 aids in the differentiation of metastatic adenocarcinoma from hepatocellular carcinoma. Cancer 1999;87:295–8.

76. Proca DM, Niemann TH, Porcell AI, et al. MOC31 immunoreactivity in primary and metastatic carcinoma of the liver. Report of findings and review of other utilized markers. Appl Immunohistochem Mol Morphol 2000;8(2):120–5.

77. Abbas A, Nikolaos V, Roland SC, et al. Hepatic angiomyolipoma: a series of six cases with emphasis on pathological-radiological correlations and unusual variants diagnosed by core needle biopsy. Int J Clin Exp Pathol 2012;5(6):512–21.

Hepatocellular Carcinoma
Histologic Subtypes

Nafis Shafizadeh, MD[a], Sanjay Kakar, MD[b],*

KEYWORDS

• Hepatocellular carcinoma • Liver • Tumor • Histologic subtypes

ABSTRACT

This review discusses the various histologic subtypes of hepatocellular carcinoma (HCC), focusing on their clinical features, pathologic features, immunohistochemical profiles, differential diagnosis, prognosis, and clinical relevance of diagnosis. The WHO recognized variants of scirrhous HCC, fibrolamellar carcinoma, combined HCC-cholangiocarcinoma (HCC-CC), sarcomatoid HCC, undifferentiated carcinoma, and lymphoepithelioma-like HCC are discussed in detail. Other subtypes including clear cell HCC, diffuse cirrhosis-like HCC, steatohepatitic HCC, transitional liver cell tumor, and CAP carcinoma are also reviewed.

SCIRRHOUS HEPATOCELLULAR CARCINOMA

Scirrhous hepatocellular carcinoma (HCC) is characterized by nests of tumor cells in a markedly fibrous stroma. There are no universally accepted criteria for the amount of fibrous stroma or the proportion of the carcinoma that should exhibit a scirrhous phenotype. The World Health Organization (WHO) definition of scirrhous HCC is vague (**Table 1**). Radiation, chemotherapy, and transarterial chemoembolization can result in marked fibrosis in conventional HCC, and such cases should not be classified as scirrhous HCC. In older literature, the term sclerosing hepatic carcinoma has been used to refer to primary hepatic carcinomas arising with marked stromal fibrosis and associated hypercalcemia.[9] Such tumors were likely a heterogeneous group, including cases of intrahepatic cholangiocarcinoma (CC). The WHO does not recognize sclerosing hepatic carcinoma as a distinct entity, and it is best to avoid the term in surgical pathology reports.

CLINICAL FEATURES

The incidence of scirrhous HCC ranges from 0.2% to 4.6%.[4] In most studies, there are no differences in demographics, presence of chronic liver disease, presence of cirrhosis, or serum alpha fetoprotein (AFP) levels in scirrhous HCC compared with conventional HCC.[3–5,7,10]

PATHOLOGIC FEATURES

Gross Features

The gross appearance of scirrhous HCC can be similar to intrahepatic CC. A capsule is typically absent and the cut surface is firm and white because of abundant fibrous stroma. Subcapsular location is common. The radiographic features of scirrhous HCC can be similar to CC. In contrast with conventional HCC, which typically shows uniform enhancement in the arterial phase and washout in the venous phase on contrast-enhanced computed tomography scan, scirrhous HCC often shows peripheral ring enhancement in the arterial phase and delayed enhancement of the central region in the venous phase.[4,5] One study showed that scirrhous HCC is frequently radiographically misdiagnosed as intrahepatic CC, combined HCC-CC, or metastatic carcinoma.[4]

Microscopic Features

In addition to abundant fibrous stroma (**Fig. 1**), other characteristic findings include absence of a fibrous capsule, no necrosis or hemorrhage, intratumoral portal tracts, and lymphocytic

[a] Department of Pathology, Woodland Hills Medical Center, 5601 De Soto Avenue, Woodland Hills, CA 91365, USA; [b] Department of Pathology, Veterans Administration Medical Center, University of California, San Francisco, 113B, 4150 Clement Street, San Francisco, CA 94121, USA
* Corresponding author.
E-mail address: sanjay.kakar@ucsf.edu

Surgical Pathology 6 (2013) 367–384
http://dx.doi.org/10.1016/j.path.2013.03.007
1875-9181/13/$ – see front matter Published by Elsevier Inc.

Table 1
Definition of scirrhous HCC in various publications

Source	Criteria
Ishak et al,[1] 2001	Trabecular HCC with abundant stroma
Matsuura et al,[2] 2005	Fibrous stroma in >25% of area of tumor microscopically, in more than half of the largest cut surface
Okamura et al,[3] 2005	Scirrhous area >50% of tumor
Kurogi et al,[4] 2006	Diffuse fibrosis in almost the entire area of largest tumor slice on gross examination
Kim et al,[5] 2009	Scirrhous area >50% of tumor
Fujii et al,[6] 2007	Abundant fibrous stroma with cords of HCC cells
Sugiki et al,[7] 2009	Almost all areas of the tumor occupied with scirrhous structures
Bosman et al,[8] 2010	Marked sinusoidal fibrosis with varying degrees of atrophy of tumor trabeculae

infiltration.[2–5,7] Clear cell change and hyaline bodies have also been reported.[4] The cytologic features are usually similar to moderately differentiated classic HCC.

Some scirrhous HCC cases are characterized by small oval cells at the periphery of the tumor cell nests. In some series, these cells are present in most scirrhous HCC cases,[10] although these have not been observed in other series.[11] These small peripheral cells may express cytokeratin 19 (CK19), neural cell adhesion molecule (NCAM or CD56), KIT (CD117), and epithelial cell adhesion molecule (EPCAM, recognized by MOC-31 antibody). Although not specific, these markers have been putatively associated with progenitor cells, and these cells have been postulated to represent cancer stem cells (discussed later). Gene expression profiling in scirrhous HCCs has shown that these tumors often express CC-like and stem cell–like genes.[12,13]

Immunohistochemical Features

Commonly used hepatocellular markers like Hep Par 1 and polyclonal carcinoembryonic antigen (CEA) are negative in more than 50% of scirrhous HCC (**Box 1**), whereas markers commonly used to identify adenocarcinoma, like CK7, CK19, and

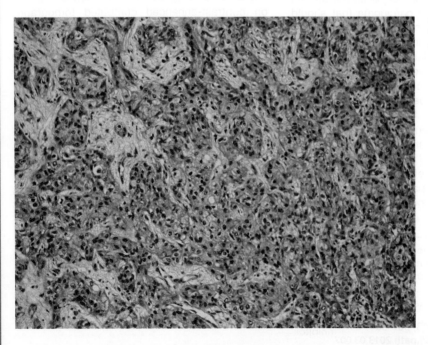

Fig. 1. Scirrhous HCC with abundant fibrous stroma.

EPCAM, are positive in nearly two-thirds of cases (**Fig. 2**A, B).[2–4] Recently described hepatocellular markers such as glypican-3 and arginase-1 are more reliable for identification of scirrhous HCC and are positive in greater than 90% of cases (see **Fig. 2**C). A sensitivity of 100% has been reported with their combined use.[11]

DIFFERENTIAL DIAGNOSIS

The distinction from fibrolamellar HCC (FLM) is based on the typical histologic features, as discussed later. The abundant stroma along with this aberrant immunophenotype can lead to an erroneous diagnosis of CC or metastatic adenocarcinoma. Glypican-3 and arginase-1 should always be included in the panel for immunohistochemical work-up of liver tumors with abundant stroma.

The distinction between scirrhous HCC and CC can have significant clinical implications for the surgical approach, chemotherapeutic regimen, and decision for transplantation. Lymph node dissection is routinely performed for CC given the high propensity for lymph node metastasis. For unresectable CCs or those with positive surgical margins after resection, the National Comprehensive Cancer Network guidelines recommend gemcitabine-based or fluoropyramidine-based chemotherapy. These drugs are ineffective in HCC, whereas sorafenib, a multikinase inhibitor, and transarterial chemoembolization are recommended.[14,15] In HCC arising in cirrhotic liver, patients are selected for transplantation using the Milan or University of California, San Francisco criteria. Although definite guidelines do not exist, most centers deny liver transplantation with a diagnosis of CC because of the high rate of recurrence. The distinction from combined HCC-CC carries the same implication because the treatment is often guided by the CC component.

PROGNOSIS

The prognosis in this variant has been variously described as worse, better, or the same as classic HCC.[2,4,5,7] Lack of uniform diagnostic criteria and small cases series may have contributed to these discrepant results. The more recent studies have argued that scirrhous HCC is a more aggressive tumor compared with classic HCC.

FIBROLAMELLAR CARCINOMA

FLM was first described by Dr Hugh Edmondson in as a liver tumor of young adults.[16] This variant was more extensively studied in 2 articles in 1980 in which the term fibrolamellar carcinoma (FLM) was coined.[17,18]

CLINICAL FEATURES

FLM is characteristically a disease of young adults with a mean age of diagnosis of 26 years.[18,19] This is in contrast with conventional HCC, for which the mean age of diagnosis is 65 years.[19] FLM is a rare tumor (representing from 1% to 8% of HCCs depending on the series) and therefore conventional HCC is still the most common primary liver tumor in young adults.[19–21] It has been reported that FLM is less common in Asia compared with the West, and no strong gender predilection has been reported.[19,22,23] Serum levels of AFP are often normal; mild increases can be seen in 10% to 15% of cases.[24] Serum B_{12} binding protein is often increased and small series suggest its use for diagnosis and recurrence.[25,26] The most distinctive feature of FLM is the absence of cirrhosis or chronic liver disease, and there are no known risk factors.[17,27] Although there have been reports of detecting hepatitis B viral DNA in neoplastic cells, it is thought that these cases are coincidental given the high worldwide prevalence of hepatitis B, and there is no definite evidence of a pathogenic role for hepatitis B.[28,29]

The mainstay of treatment is aggressive surgical resection, with the preferred treatment being complete excision of the affected lobe. Lymph node involvement has been reported in up to 70% of cases, and hence regional lymph node dissection is often performed.[21,30,31] Liver transplantation is sometimes performed when resection is not possible. In the absence of surgical resection, median survival is 1 year.[31] Limited studies on adjuvant therapy have not shown enhanced survival with chemotherapeutic agents.[20,22]

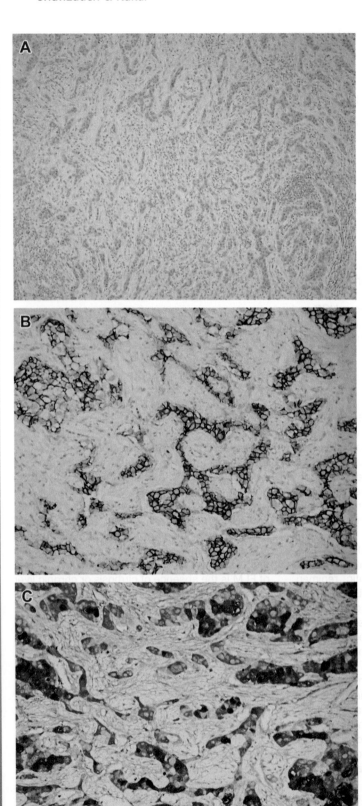

Fig. 2. Scirrhous HCC with negative Hep Par 1 (*A*), strong expression of EPCAM (*B*), and positive arginase-1 (*C*).

MORPHOLOGIC FEATURES

Gross Features

FLMs are large tan-white tumors occurring in non-cirrhotic livers. Although there are rare reports of FLM in cirrhotic livers, the diagnosis of FLM in the presence of cirrhosis should be reconsidered. FLMs are significantly larger on presentation than conventional HCC.[24,32,33] They also often show a central scar with calcifications, which can suggest the diagnosis radiographically.[23]

Microscopic Features

FLM is defined by a triad of histologic features (Fig. 3). The typical clinicopathologic associations of FLM are observed if these criteria are strictly

Fig. 3. The characteristic triad of histologic features of FLM: Lamellar fibrous stroma (A), abundant eosinophilic granular cytoplasm, and a single prominent nucleolus (B).

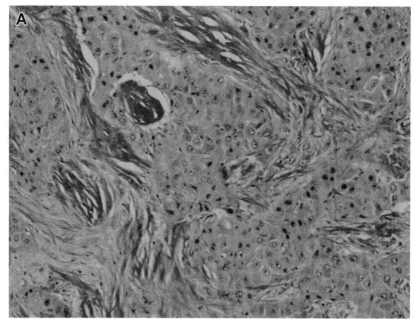

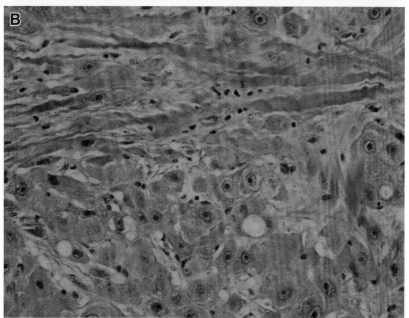

applied and the diagnosis reserved for cases that satisfy all three criteria (**Box 2**).

1. Large polygonal tumor cells with abundant eosinophilic granular cytoplasm. The cytoplasmic morphology is caused by abundant mitochondria.[34] Recent studies also suggest lysosomal or endosomal cytoplasmic accumulations.[35] Other cytoplasmic features that can be seen include a ground-glass appearance, oval eosinophilic inclusions known as pale bodies (**Fig. 4**), and PASD-positive cytoplasmic globules. These cytoplasmic features are not necessary for the diagnosis, and can also be seen in conventional HCC.
2. Prominent eosinophilic macronucleoli. These large nucleoli often reside in a nucleus with vesicular chromatin.
3. Plate-like stacks of collagen (ie, lamellar fibrosis). This pattern of fibrosis can be patchy but is usually present in at least half of the tumor.

Other morphologic features of FLM include reduced mitotic activity, canalicular bile plugs with associated copper deposition, and nuclear enlargement with smudgy chromatin giving an appearance of degenerative atypia.[33] A clear cell variant of FLM has been described.[36]

FLM occasionally forms pseudoacinar structures with mucin, giving an appearance of biliary differentiation, and they have been mistakenly characterized as mixed FLM-CC in some series.[37] These tumors do not show typical morphology of CC and are considered morphologic variants of FLM. Rare cases of true combined tumors with well-defined FLM and CC can occur. Some tumors are comprised of both FLM and conventional HCC components.[38] Pure FLMs occur in a younger age group, have decreased levels of serum AFP, have a higher incidence of nodal disease, and have a prolonged survival compared with mixed FLM-HCC, suggesting that mixed FLM-HCC are more related to conventional HCC.[38]

Immunohistochemical Features

FLMs are positive for hepatocellular markers, including Hep Par 1, polyclonal CEA (canalicular staining), and arginase-1. AFP immunoreactivity is rare,[39] and positivity for glypican-3 varies from 18% to 64%.[40–44] Cytokeratin 7 (CK7) is often positive, ranging from 80% to 100%, compared with only 20% to 30% of conventional HCC.[40,41,44,45] Markers for neuroendocrine differentiation, such as nonspecific enolase and chromogranin, can be positive.[46,47] A recent study showed the high sensitivity of CD68, with positivity seen in 97% of FLM cases. However, CD68 was not very specific, with positivity seen in 25% of HCC without cirrhosis and in 11% of HCC with cirrhosis.[35]

Expression of stem cell–associated markers such as EPCAM, NCAM, CD133, and CD44 has been reported in some cases of FLM.[44,48] These findings, along with focal glandular differentiation in some cases and a high frequency of CK7 expression, have led to the hypothesis that FLM may have stem cell–like properties.

DIFFERENTIAL DIAGNOSIS

Prominent stromal fibrosis and frequent CK7 expression in scirrhous HCC can mimic FLM. The typical cytologic features of FLM are not seen in scirrhous HCC, and the fibrosis in most cases does not have lamellar characteristics.

The pseudoacinar structures, mucin, and CK7 positivity in FLM can be mistaken for CC or metastatic adenocarcinoma, whereas occasional positivity for neuroendocrine markers can lead to an erroneous diagnosis of neuroendocrine carcinoma. Expression of hepatocellular markers and strict adherence to the morphologic triad of histologic features helps in establishing the correct diagnosis.

PROGNOSIS

When FLM was first described as a distinct entity, initial studies showed that it had a better prognosis

---

Box 2
FLM

FLM: practical points

- Typically occurs in young adults
- No history of chronic liver disease or cirrhosis
- Lymph node involvement more common than conventional HCC
- Central scar may be present
- Histologic triad: lamellar fibrosis, eosinophilic granular cytoplasm, prominent nucleolus
- Focal glandular architecture and mucin can be present
- CK7 (often) and neuroendocrine markers (occasional) can be positive
- Aggressive tumor with 5-year survival similar to conventional HCC arising in noncirrhotic liver

Fig. 4. Pale bodies in FLM, which are cytoplasmic accumulations of fibrinogen and can also be observed in conventional HCC.

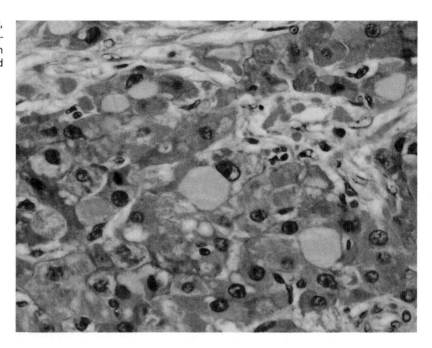

compared with conventional HCC, and a misconception grew that it was an indolent tumor.[18,27,32,33,49] However, FLM is an aggressive tumor that can present with surgically unresectable extrahepatic disease. Lymph node and peritoneal metastases are more common than in conventional HCC, with lymph node involvement being reported in up to 70% of cases.[18,21,30,31] Recent studies have shown that prognosis in FLM is similar to conventional HCC occurring in noncirrhotic liver.[24] The 5-year survival in FLM is 50% to 60% in most series, with surgical resectability being the most important prognostic factor.[18,24,27,49]

COMBINED HCC-CC

This tumor was first described by H. Gideon Wells in 1903, when he described a single autopsy report of a liver with alcoholic cirrhosis and a carcinoma arising from both the bile ducts and from the hepatic cells.[50] The current WHO definition of a combined HCC-CC is a tumor containing unequivocal, intimately mixed elements of both HCC and CC.[8] Separate nodules comprising HCC and CC adjacent to each other in the same liver (collision tumor) are not considered combined HCC-CC. The conflicting data regarding combined HCC-CC in the literature is caused by the use of different definitions, and categorization of collision tumors and FLM with focal mucin as combined HCC-CCs.[37,51]

Two subtypes of combined HCC-CC are recognized in the current WHO scheme:

1. Classic type
2. Combined HCC-CC with stem cell features

COMBINED HCC-CC, CLASSIC TYPE

Clinical Features

In most studies, the clinical features of HCC-CC such as age, gender, viral hepatitis status, and cirrhosis are similar to HCC rather than CC.[52–55] Several studies have shown an increased rate of lymph node metastasis in HCC-CC compared with HCC that is similar to that of CC.[52,56] There have been conflicting results regarding prognosis, with some studies showing a worse prognosis than for both HCC and CC, and others showing an intermediate prognosis between HCC and CC.[52–57]

Pathologic Features

This tumor contains areas of typical HCC and typical CC, and may have foci of intermediate morphology at the interface (**Box 3**, **Figs. 5–8**). The HCC component may have varying degrees of differentiation and often shows the typical trabecular architecture. Confirmation of the hepatocellular component is imperative for the diagnosis and can be achieved by immunohistochemistry or albumin in situ hybridization.[37,58,59] Biliary differentiation is recognized by discrete

---

Box 3
Combined HCC-CC, classic subtype

Combined HCC-CC, classic subtype: practical points

- Both components seen in the same tumor nodule

- Clinical features similar to HCC

- Lymph node metastasis and aggressive behavior similar to CC

- Hepatocellular component: confirm with markers like Hep Par 1 and arginase-1

- CC component: discrete gland formation and/or mucin

- Positivity for CK7, CK19, and MOC-31 can be seen in HCC and does not by itself constitute evidence of CC component

- Transitional areas with overlapping features of HCC and CC are common

- Because of treatment implications, criteria should be strictly applied for diagnosis

---

gland formation, desmoplastic stroma, and/or mucin production. This component usually stains with CK7, CK19, and MOC-31; however, these markers also stain a subset of HCCs and are not specific for biliary differentiation.[58–60]

Differential Diagnosis

The implications of this diagnosis can be significant because the surgical approach, chemotherapeutic regimen, and option for transplantation may be significantly affected by the CC component. There is an increased likelihood of lymph node metastasis compared with conventional HCC.[52,56] Therefore, a preoperative diagnosis of HCC-CC on a core biopsy may alter the surgical management and prompt a hilar lymph node dissection.[61] There are limited data on the role of transplantation, with a single small case series showing long-term survival in only 1 of 3 patients.[62] Although there are no definite guidelines, it is likely that a diagnosis of combined HCC-CC precludes the patient from transplantation. Fluoropyrimidine-based or gemcitabine-based chemotherapy may be used in these cases targeting the CC component.

It is therefore important to use strict criteria for the diagnosis of both HCC and CC components. The HCC component must be confirmed by immunohistochemistry, whereas discrete well-formed glands or mucin must be identified for the CC component. CC should not be diagnosed based on pseudoglandular architecture or expression of CK7/CK19/MOC-31 in a tumor that otherwise shows features of HCC.

HCC-CC WITH STEM CELL FEATURES

Most combined HCC-CCs show transitional areas where tumor cells show overlap of hepatocellular

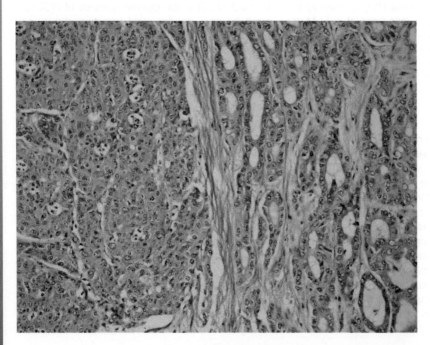

Fig. 5. Combined HCC-CC, classic type. Trabecular pattern of HCC (*left*) with discrete glandular areas of CC (*right*).

Fig. 6. Combined HCC-CC, classic type. HCC portion is highlighted by positive staining with arginase-1.

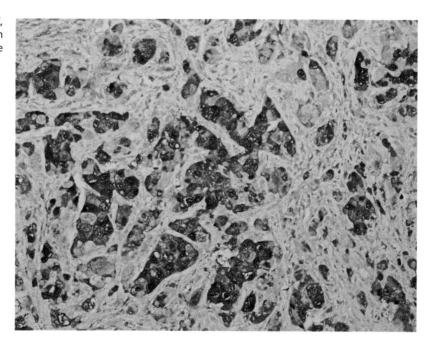

and biliary features at both the morphologic and immunohistochemical level. In some tumors, these transitional areas predominate and have been referred to as intermediate carcinomas. The current WHO scheme refers to these tumors as combined HCC-CC with stem cell features (**Box 4, Table 2**). Stem cell or progenitor cell morphologic features include small size, oval shape, hyperchromatic nuclei, scant cytoplasm, and no or mild cytologic atypia; and, immunohistochemically, these cells can be positive for CK19, MOC-31, and a variety of putative stem cell markers like NCAM, KIT, and CD133. These cells are reminiscent of hepatic progenitor cells normally found in

Fig. 7. Combined HCC-CC, classic type. CC area with gland formation and strong staining for CK19 (*left*); weaker CK19 staining is seen in the HCC portion (*right*).

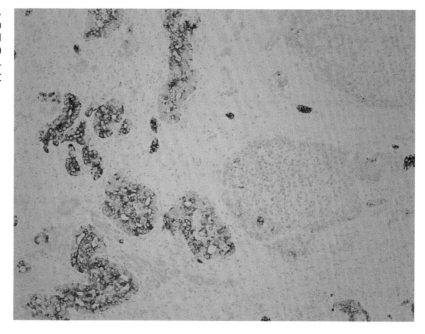

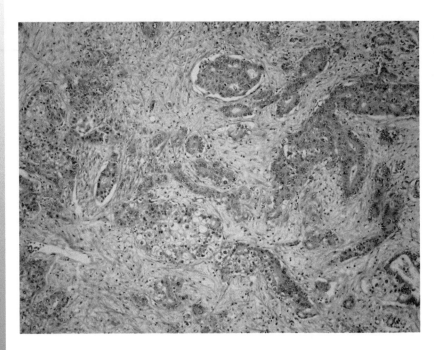

Fig. 8. Combined HCC-CC, classic type. Transitional area between HCC and CC demonstrating features of both elements.

the canals of Hering, and have been proposed to be cancer stem cells. Although the following 3 subtypes have been proposed by the WHO, they are not considered to be distinct entities because it is unclear whether biological or clinical differences exist between them.

Box 4
Combined HCC-CC, stem cell features

Combined HCC-CC, stem cell features: practical points
- Areas with morphologic resemblance to stem cell/progenitor cells predominate

- Morphologic features: small size, oval shape, scant cytoplasm, high N/C ratio, no or mild cytologic atypia; abundant fibrous stroma is common

- Immunohistochemical features: variable positive staining for CK19, EPCAM, KIT, CD56, CD133

- WHO 2010 proposes 3 morphologic subtypes: typical, intermediate, and cholangiolocellular

- Initial studies suggest an aggressive behavior, but there is insufficient information for definite conclusions

- Similar to the classic subtype, typical HCC and CC components must be present

---

The typical subtype is similar to scirrhous HCC except that it contains peripheral clusters of small cells with high N/C ratios similar to hepatic progenitor cells (**Fig. 9**). These cells are positive for many of the hepatic stem cell markers including CK7, CK19, NCAM, and EPCAM. It is of great historical interest that Edmondson and Steiner,[16] in their 1954 article describing and classifying 100 cases of primary liver carcinoma (one of the first thorough histologic classifications and discussions of liver carcinoma involving a large series of cases) recognized and described the small peripheral oval cells seen in some cases of combined HCC-CC (the reader is referred to their article for a photomicrograph, and its caption, as evidence of their recognition).[16] They referred to these cells as the "primitive peripheral layer," and even postulated that they "probably [have] the potentiality of differentiating into adenocarcinoma similar to that derived from intrahepatic bile ducts". In the intermediate cell subtype, the tumor is nearly entirely composed of the areas of transition between hepatocellular and biliary differentiation (**Fig. 10**). These tumors stain with both hepatocellular and biliary markers and are often positive for KIT. The cholangiolocellular subtype (which was formerly a subtype of CC) is a tumor with tubular or cord-like anastomosing architecture, often referred to as an antler-like pattern, set in an abundant fibrous stroma (**Fig. 11**). The individual cells are small with high N/C ratios and

Table 2
Three subtypes of combined HCC-CC with stem cell features

	Combined HCC-CC with Stem Cell Features, Typical Subtype[10,63]	Combined HCC-CC with Stem Cell Features, Intermediate Cell Subtype[64]	Combined HCC-CC with Stem Cell Features, Cholangiolocellular Subtype[65]

Morphology	a. Solid nests of mature-appearing hepatocytes, may have clear cytoplasm
	b. Peripheral clusters of small cells with high N/C ratio and hyperchromatic nuclei
	c. Scirrhous stroma can be present
		a. Solid nests, strands, trabeculae in scirrhous stroma
		b. Intermediate between hepatocytes and cholangiocytes
		  i. Small oval cells
		  ii. Hyperchromatic nuclei
		  iii. Scant cytoplasm
		c. Elongated ill-defined gland-like structures, no definite glands or mucin
			a. Small cells with high N/C ratio
			b. Tubular, cord-like, anastomosing pattern (antler-like)
			c. Scirrhous stroma
			d. Atypia mild, mucin absent
			e. Conventional HCC-like and CC-like areas at the periphery

Immunohistochemistry	Small cells often positive for K7, K19, CD56, MOC-31 (EPCAM)	a. Simultaneous staining with HCC and adenocarcinoma markers b. KIT often positive	Often positive for K19, KIT, NCAM, MOC-31 (EPCAM)

hyperchromatic oval nuclei. The periphery of these tumors often shows more conventional HCC-like and/or CC-like morphologies with areas of transition. They are CK7, CK19, KIT, and NCAM positive. Similar to the classic subtype of combined HCC-CC, discrete components of HCC and CC must be identified in addition to the stem cell component before the tumor is categorized as combined HCC-CC with stem cell features.

Fig. 9. Combined HCC-CC, stem cell features, typical subtype. Islands of tumor cells in an abundant fibrous stroma resembling scirrhous HCC with small uniform round to oval cells at the periphery of the tumor cells nests.

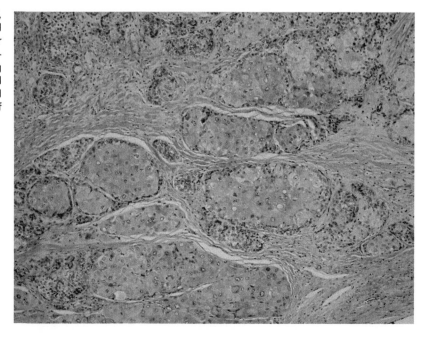

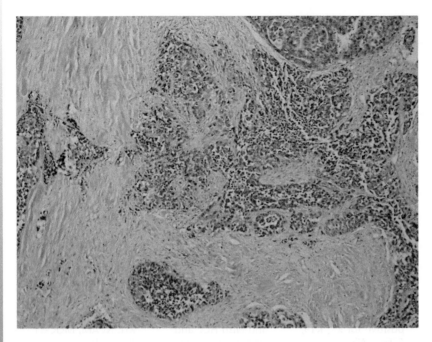

Fig. 10. Combined HCC-CC, stem cell features, intermediate subtype. Trabeculae composed of cells with hyperchromatic nuclei and scanty cytoplasm embedded in a fibrous stroma. A portion of typical HCC is also present (*upper right*).

Sarcomatoid HCC

This subtype is partially or fully composed of malignant spindle cells with or without evidence of heterologous differentiation (Fig. 12). When the tumor is entirely composed of malignant spindle cells, clinical history and immunohistochemistry may be the sole mechanisms to recognize the hepatocellular nature of the malignancy. Various types of heterologous elements have been reported, including rhabdoid, osteoid, and chondroid differentiation.[66–68] The data on sarcomatoid HCC are limited to case reports and small series and the incidence has been suggested to be between 1.8% and 3.9% of HCCs.[69,70] Lower

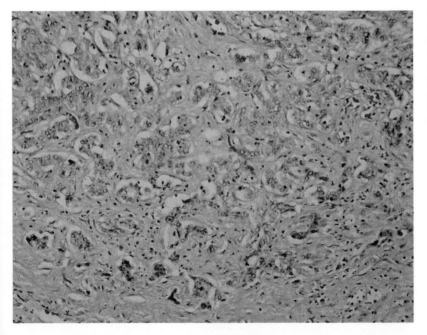

Fig. 11. Combined HCC-CC, stem cell features, cholangiolocellular subtype. Anastomosing elongated ductules (antler-like pattern) composed of small uniform cells embedded in a fibrous stroma.

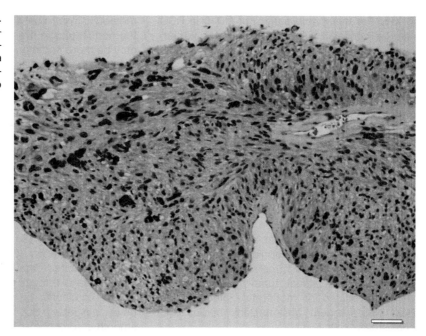

Fig. 12. Sarcomatoid HCC. The morphology is indistinguishable from a sarcoma; the presence of a component of conventional HCC is necessary to make the diagnosis.

serum AFP, higher incidence of extrahepatic disease, and a worse prognosis compared with conventional HCC have been reported.[69,70] Hepatocellular markers are typically negative in the malignant spindle cell component, whereas keratin positivity has been observed in 23% to 63% of cases.[69,70]

Undifferentiated Carcinoma

Histologic grading is based on tumor differentiation, and a system of grading was first described by Edmondson and Steiner in 1954.[16] Well-differentiated HCCs are small tumors (less than 2 cm) and closely recapitulate liver parenchyma in a trabecular or pseudoglandular architecture. Tumors that are moderately differentiated are typically greater than 3 cm and have abundant eosinophilic cytoplasm and distinct nucleoli. HCC that is poorly differentiated grows in a solid or trabecular pattern and often shows high N/C ratios and marked pleomorphism. Undifferentiated carcinoma is defined as a tumor that is primary to the liver but can only be diagnosed as carcinoma from immunohistochemistry, and cannot be further classified. Several studies have shown that tumor differentiation predicts prognosis and recurrence.[71–73] Undifferentiated carcinomas are thought to have a worse prognosis compared with conventional HCC.[1]

Lymphoepithelioma-like HCC

This is an extremely rare tumor, and is characterized by pleomorphic tumor cells set in a dense lymphoid stroma. Cases with intense lymphocytic infiltration should be classified into this category, whereas tumors with a mild to moderate increase in lymphocytes are regarded as conventional HCC. Most of the infiltrating lymphocytes are T cells. A small number of cases have been reported, and it is difficult to draw clinicopathologic conclusions regarding this entity.[74–77] Most cases have been Epstein-Barr virus (EBV) negative by in situ hybridization or polymerase chain reaction; EBV positivity has been described in 1 study.[77]

Other Subtypes

Clear cell HCC is not considered a histologic subtype of HCC and clear cells can be seen in any of the subtypes described in this article. It can be confused with other metastatic clear cell neoplasms, most notably clear cell renal cell carcinoma (RCC). Hepatocellular markers like Hep Par 1, polyclonal CEA (canalicular pattern), and arginase-1 are positive in HCC but negative in RCC.[78,79] Transcription factors PAX-2 and PAX-8 have high sensitivity and specificity for RCC and are negative in HCC.[80,81] RCC antigen and CD10 are less sensitive for RCC, but can increase sensitivity when used in combination with PAX-2 or

PAX-8. The membrane pattern of CD10 in RCC can be confused with the canalicular pattern seen in HCC.[82,83] Keratin subtypes are not helpful because both RCC and HCC are positive for CAM 5.2 and are typically negative for both CK7 and CK20. Clear cell HCC has been associated with hepatitis C infection, a low rate of vascular invasion, and a better prognosis.[84]

Diffuse cirrhosis-like HCC has a characteristic appearance on imaging and gross examination, but does not have distinctive histologic features and is not a WHO-recognized subtype. The tumor forms multiple small nodules that are intimately admixed with the nodules of a cirrhotic liver. It is often diagnosed on the explant specimen at the time of transplantation, because it is undetected radiographically or clinically. Most patients have no, or minimal, increase in AFP. The individual tumor nodules show well-differentiated or moderately differentiated HCC with frequent Mallory-Denk bodies and cholestasis.[85]

Steatohepatitic HCC is a recently described variant in which the morphologic findings of steatohepatitis are seen in the tumor (Fig. 13): steatosis, ballooning, Mallory-Denk bodies, and pericellular fibrosis.[86] In well-differentiated cases, the findings can be mistaken for steatohepatitis and the tumor can be overlooked. Prominent intratumoral fibrosis and infiltrative borders are common findings. The patients often have metabolic syndrome–associated risk factors and the nonneoplastic liver shows steatohepatitis. It may be more common in nonalcoholic steatohepatitis than in alcoholic liver disease.[87] Similar tumors can occur in patients without metabolic risk factors and with no evidence of steatohepatitis in nonneoplastic liver. Although data are still limited on this histologic variant, one study has shown no difference in survival or metastasis compared with conventional HCC.[88]

Transitional liver cell tumor is a term used to describe rare cases with morphologic features overlapping between HCC and hepatoblastoma.[89] The tumor occurs in older children and adolescents (5–18 years old). Most tumors are AFP positive, CK19 negative, and epithelial membrane antigen (EMA) negative. Although there are limited data on this subtype, the clinical course is thought to be aggressive.

CAP carcinoma is an acronym coined for a newly described HCC variant characterized by smooth chromophobic cytoplasm, abrupt nuclear anaplasia (small clusters of tumor cells with marked nuclear anaplasia in a background of tumor cells with bland nuclear cytology), and scattered microscopic pseudocysts.[90] By telomere-specific fluorescent in situ hybridization, these tumors showed alternative lengthening of telomeres (ALT), a finding not typically seen in conventional HCC. Further studies are required to establish it as a distinct clinicopathologic entity.

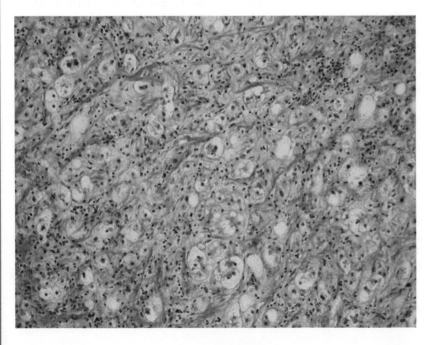

Fig. 13. Steatohepatitic HCC. The tumor cells show fat, ballooning, and Mallory hyaline. (*Courtesy of* Dr Linda Ferrell, MD, University of CA, San Francisco.)

REFERENCES

1. Ishak KG, Goodman ZD, Stocker JT. Tumors of the liver and intrahepatic bile ducts. Washington, DC: Armed Forces Institute of Pathology; 2001.
2. Matsuura S, Aishima S, Taguchi K, et al. 'Scirrhous' type hepatocellular carcinomas: a special reference to expression of cytokeratin 7 and hepatocyte paraffin 1. Histopathology 2005;47:382–90.
3. Okamura N, Yoshida M, Shibuya A, et al. Cellular and stromal characteristics in the scirrhous hepatocellular carcinoma: comparison with hepatocellular carcinomas and intrahepatic cholangiocarcinomas. Pathol Int 2005;55:724–31.
4. Kurogi M, Nakashima O, Miyaaki H, et al. Clinicopathological study of scirrhous hepatocellular carcinoma. J Gastroenterol Hepatol 2006;21:1470–7.
5. Kim SH, Lim HK, Lee WJ, et al. Scirrhous hepatocellular carcinoma: comparison with usual hepatocellular carcinoma based on CT-pathologic features and long-term results after curative resection. Eur J Radiol 2009;69:123–30.
6. Fujii T, Zen Y, Nakanuma Y. Minute scirrhous hepatocellular carcinomas undergoing different carcinogenetic processes. Pathol Int 2007;57:443–8.
7. Sugiki T, Yamamoto M, Taka K, et al. Specific characteristics of scirrhous hepatocellular carcinoma. Hepatogastroenterology 2009;56:1086–9.
8. Bosman FT, Carneiro F, Hruban RH, et al. WHO Classification of tumours of the digestive system. Lyon (France): World Health Organization Press; 2010.
9. Omata M, Peters RL, Tatter D. Sclerosing hepatic carcinoma: relationship to hypercalcemia. Liver 1981;1:33–49.
10. Fujii T, Zen Y, Harada K, et al. Participation of liver cancer stem/progenitor cells in tumorigenesis of scirrhous hepatocellular carcinoma–human and cell culture study. Hum Pathol 2008;39:1185–96.
11. Krings G, Ramachandran R, Jain D, et al. Immunohistochemical pitfalls and the importance of glypican 3 and arginase in the diagnosis of scirrhous hepatocellular carcinoma. Mod Pathol 2013:243.
12. Seok JY, Na DC, Woo HG, et al. A fibrous stromal component in hepatocellular carcinoma reveals a cholangiocarcinoma-like gene expression trait and epithelial-mesenchymal transition. Hepatology 2012;55:1776–86.
13. Woo HG, Lee JH, Yoon JH, et al. Identification of a cholangiocarcinoma-like gene expression trait in hepatocellular carcinoma. Cancer Res 2010;70:3034–41.
14. Choi SB, Kim KS, Choi JY, et al. The prognosis and survival outcome of intrahepatic cholangiocarcinoma following surgical resection: association of lymph node metastasis and lymph node dissection with survival. Ann Surg Oncol 2009;16:3048–56.
15. Morise Z, Sugioka A, Tokoro T, et al. Surgery and chemotherapy for intrahepatic cholangiocarcinoma. World J Hepatol 2010;2:58–64.
16. Edmondson HA, Steiner PE. Primary carcinoma of the liver: a study of 100 cases among 48,900 necropsies. Cancer 1954;7:462–503.
17. Berman MM, Libbey NP, Foster JH. Hepatocellular carcinoma. Polygonal cell type with fibrous stroma–an atypical variant with a favorable prognosis. Cancer 1980;46:1448–55.
18. Craig JR, Peters RL, Edmondson HA, et al. Fibrolamellar carcinoma of the liver: a tumor of adolescents and young adults with distinctive clinico-pathologic features. Cancer 1980;46:372–9.
19. El-Serag HB, Davila JA. Is fibrolamellar carcinoma different from hepatocellular carcinoma? A US population-based study. Hepatology 2004;39:798–803.
20. Pinna AD, Iwatsuki S, Lee RG, et al. Treatment of fibrolamellar hepatoma with subtotal hepatectomy or transplantation. Hepatology 1997;26:877–83.
21. Stevens WR, Johnson CD, Stephens DH, et al. Fibrolamellar hepatocellular carcinoma: stage at presentation and results of aggressive surgical management. AJR Am J Roentgenol 1995;164:1153–8.
22. El-Gazzaz G, Wong W, El-Hadary MK, et al. Outcome of liver resection and transplantation for fibrolamellar hepatocellular carcinoma. Transpl Int 2000;13(Suppl 1):S406–9.
23. McLarney JK, Rucker PT, Bender GN, et al. Fibrolamellar carcinoma of the liver: radiologic-pathologic correlation. Radiographics 1999;19:453–71.
24. Kakar S, Burgart LJ, Batts KP, et al. Clinicopathologic features and survival in fibrolamellar carcinoma: comparison with conventional hepatocellular carcinoma with and without cirrhosis. Mod Pathol 2005;18:1417–23.
25. Lildballe DL, Nguyen KQ, Poulsen SS, et al. Haptocorrin as marker of disease progression in fibrolamellar hepatocellular carcinoma. Eur J Surg Oncol 2011;37:72–9.
26. Paradinas FJ, Melia WM, Wilkinson ML, et al. High serum vitamin B_{12} binding capacity as a marker of the fibrolamellar variant of hepatocellular carcinoma. Br Med J (Clin Res Ed) 1982;285:840–2.
27. Hodgson HJ. Fibrolamellar cancer of the liver. J Hepatol 1987;5:241–7.
28. Chang YC, Dai YC, Chow NH. Fibrolamellar hepatocellular carcinoma with a recurrence of classic hepatocellular carcinoma: a case report and review of Oriental cases. Hepatogastroenterology 2003;50:1637–40.
29. Davison FD, Fagan EA, Portmann B, et al. HBV-DNA sequences in tumor and nontumor tissue

in a patient with the fibrolamellar variant of hepatocellular carcinoma. Hepatology 1990;12: 676–9.

30. Maniaci V, Davidson BR, Rolles K, et al. Fibrolamellar hepatocellular carcinoma: prolonged survival with multimodality therapy. Eur J Surg Oncol 2009;35:617–21.

31. Stipa F, Yoon SS, Liau KH, et al. Outcome of patients with fibrolamellar hepatocellular carcinoma. Cancer 2006;106:1331–8.

32. Berman MA, Burnham JA, Sheahan DG. Fibrolamellar carcinoma of the liver: an immunohistochemical study of nineteen cases and a review of the literature. Hum Pathol 1988;19:784–94.

33. Farhi DC, Shikes RH, Murari PJ, et al. Hepatocellular carcinoma in young people. Cancer 1983;52: 1516–25.

34. Farhi DC, Shikes RH, Silverberg SG. Ultrastructure of fibrolamellar oncocytic hepatoma. Cancer 1982; 50:702–9.

35. Ross HM, Daniel HD, Vivekanandan P, et al. Fibrolamellar carcinomas are positive for CD68. Mod Pathol 2011;24:390–5.

36. Cheuk W, Chan JK. Clear cell variant of fibrolamellar carcinoma of the liver. Arch Pathol Lab Med 2001;125:1235–8.

37. Goodman ZD, Ishak KG, Langloss JM, et al. Combined hepatocellular-cholangiocarcinoma. A histologic and immunohistochemical study. Cancer 1985;55:124–35.

38. Malouf GG, Brugieres L, Le Deley MC, et al. Pure and mixed fibrolamellar hepatocellular carcinomas differ in natural history and prognosis after complete surgical resection. Cancer 2012;118(20): 4981–90.

39. Caballero T, Aneiros J, Lopez-Caballero J, et al. Fibrolamellar hepatocellular carcinoma. An immunohistochemical and ultrastructural study. Histopathology 1985;9:445–56.

40. Abdul-Al HM, Wang G, Makhlouf HR, et al. Fibrolamellar hepatocellular carcinoma: an immunohistochemical comparison with conventional hepatocellular carcinoma. Int J Surg Pathol 2010;18: 313–8.

41. Patonai A, Erdelyi-Belle B, Korompay A, et al. Claudins and tricellulin in fibrolamellar hepatocellular carcinoma. Virchows Arch 2011;458:679–88.

42. Shafizadeh N, Ferrell LD, Kakar S. Utility and limitations of glypican-3 expression for the diagnosis of hepatocellular carcinoma at both ends of the differentiation spectrum. Mod Pathol 2008;21:1011–8.

43. Wang XY, Degos F, Dubois S, et al. Glypican-3 expression in hepatocellular tumors: diagnostic value for preneoplastic lesions and hepatocellular carcinomas. Hum Pathol 2006;37:1435–41.

44. Ward SC, Huang J, Tickoo SK, et al. Fibrolamellar carcinoma of the liver exhibits immunohistochemical evidence of both hepatocyte and bile duct differentiation. Mod Pathol 2010;23:1180–90.

45. Klein WM, Molmenti EP, Colombani PM, et al. Primary liver carcinoma arising in people younger than 30 years. Am J Clin Pathol 2005;124: 512–8.

46. Gornicka B, Ziarkiewicz-Wroblewska B, Wroblewski T, et al. Carcinoma, a fibrolamellar variant–immunohistochemical analysis of 4 cases. Hepatogastroenterology 2005;52:519–23.

47. Wang JH, Dhillon AP, Sankey EA, et al. 'Neuroendocrine' differentiation in primary neoplasms of the liver. J Pathol 1991;163:61–7.

48. Wilczek E, Szparecki G, Lukasik D, et al. Loss of the orphan nuclear receptor SHP is more pronounced in fibrolamellar carcinoma than in typical hepatocellular carcinoma. PLoS One 2012;7: e30944.

49. Lack EE, Neave C, Vawter GF. Hepatocellular carcinoma. Review of 32 cases in childhood and adolescence. Cancer 1983;52:1510–5.

50. Wells H. Primary carcinoma of the liver. Am J Med Sci 1903;126:403–17.

51. Allen RA, Lisa JR. Combined liver cell and bile duct carcinoma. Am J Pathol 1949;25:647–55.

52. Lee WS, Lee KW, Heo JS, et al. Comparison of combined hepatocellular and cholangiocarcinoma with hepatocellular carcinoma and intrahepatic cholangiocarcinoma. Surg Today 2006;36: 892–7.

53. Liu CL, Fan ST, Lo CM, et al. Hepatic resection for combined hepatocellular and cholangiocarcinoma. Arch Surg 2003;138:86–90.

54. Tang D, Nagano H, Nakamura M, et al. Clinical and pathological features of Allen's type C classification of resected combined hepatocellular and cholangiocarcinoma: a comparative study with hepatocellular carcinoma and cholangiocellular carcinoma. J Gastrointest Surg 2006;10:987–98.

55. Yano Y, Yamamoto J, Kosuge T, et al. Combined hepatocellular and cholangiocarcinoma: a clinicopathologic study of 26 resected cases. Jpn J Clin Oncol 2003;33:283–7.

56. Zuo HQ, Yan LN, Zeng Y, et al. Clinicopathological characteristics of 15 patients with combined hepatocellular carcinoma and cholangiocarcinoma. Hepatobiliary Pancreat Dis Int 2007;6:161–5.

57. Jarnagin WR, Weber S, Tickoo SK, et al. Combined hepatocellular and cholangiocarcinoma: demographic, clinical, and prognostic factors. Cancer 2002;94:2040–6.

58. Shirakawa H, Kuronuma T, Nishimura Y, et al. Glypican-3 is a useful diagnostic marker for a component of hepatocellular carcinoma in human liver cancer. Int J Oncol 2009;34:649–56.

59. Tickoo SK, Zee SY, Obiekwe S, et al. Combined hepatocellular-cholangiocarcinoma: a histopathologic,

immunohistochemical, and in situ hybridization study. Am J Surg Pathol 2002;26:989–97.

60. Taguchi J, Nakashima O, Tanaka M, et al. A clinicopathological study on combined hepatocellular and cholangiocarcinoma. J Gastroenterol Hepatol 1996;11:758–64.

61. Kassahun WT, Hauss J. Management of combined hepatocellular and cholangiocarcinoma. Int J Clin Pract 2008;62:1271–8.

62. Maganty K, Levi D, Moon J, et al. Combined hepatocellular carcinoma and intrahepatic cholangiocarcinoma: outcome after liver transplantation. Dig Dis Sci 2010;55:3597–601.

63. Theise ND, Yao JL, Harada K, et al. Hepatic 'stem cell' malignancies in adults: four cases. Histopathology 2003;43:263–71.

64. Kim H, Park C, Han KH, et al. Primary liver carcinoma of intermediate (hepatocyte-cholangiocyte) phenotype. J Hepatol 2004;40:298–304.

65. Komuta M, Spee B, Vander BS, et al. Clinicopathological study on cholangiolocellular carcinoma suggesting hepatic progenitor cell origin. Hepatology 2008;47:1544–56.

66. Akasofu M, Kawahara E, Kaji K, et al. Sarcomatoid hepatocellular-carcinoma showing rhabdomyoblastic differentiation in the adult cirrhotic liver. Virchows Arch 1999;434:511–5.

67. Chen CY, Hsueh YT, Lan TY, et al. Pelvic skeletal metastasis of hepatocellular carcinoma with sarcomatous change: a case report. Diagn Pathol 2010; 5:33.

68. Lao XM, Chen DY, Zhang YQ, et al. Primary carcinosarcoma of the liver: clinicopathologic features of 5 cases and a review of the literature. Am J Surg Pathol 2007;31:817–26.

69. Kakizoe S, Kojiro M, Nakashima T. Hepatocellular carcinoma with sarcomatous change. Clinicopathologic and immunohistochemical studies of 14 autopsy cases. Cancer 1987;59:310–6.

70. Maeda T, Adachi E, Kajiyama K, et al. Spindle cell hepatocellular carcinoma. A clinicopathologic and immunohistochemical analysis of 15 cases. Cancer 1996;77:51–7.

71. Lauwers GY, Terris B, Balis UJ, et al. Prognostic histologic indicators of curatively resected hepatocellular carcinomas: a multi-institutional analysis of 425 patients with definition of a histologic prognostic index. Am J Surg Pathol 2002; 26:25–34.

72. Roayaie S, Schwartz JD, Sung MW, et al. Recurrence of hepatocellular carcinoma after liver transplant: patterns and prognosis. Liver Transpl 2004; 10:534–40.

73. Zavaglia C, De CL, Alberti AB, et al. Predictors of long-term survival after liver transplantation for hepatocellular carcinoma. Am J Gastroenterol 2005; 100:2708–16.

74. Chen CJ, Jeng LB, Huang SF. Lymphoepithelioma-like hepatocellular carcinoma. Chang Gung Med J 2007;30:172–7.

75. Emile JF, Adam R, Sebagh M, et al. Hepatocellular carcinoma with lymphoid stroma: a tumour with good prognosis after liver transplantation. Histopathology 2000;37:523–9.

76. Nemolato S, Fanni D, Naccarato AG, et al. Lymphoepithelioma-like hepatocellular carcinoma: a case report and a review of the literature. World J Gastroenterol 2008;14:4694–6.

77. Si MW, Thorson JA, Lauwers GY, et al. Hepatocellular lymphoepithelioma-like carcinoma associated with Epstein Barr virus: a hitherto unrecognized entity. Diagn Mol Pathol 2004;13:183–9.

78. Murakata LA, Ishak KG, Nzeako UC. Clear cell carcinoma of the liver: a comparative immunohistochemical study with renal clear cell carcinoma. Mod Pathol 2000;13:874–81.

79. Yan BC, Gong C, Song J, et al. Arginase-1: a new immunohistochemical marker of hepatocytes and hepatocellular neoplasms. Am J Surg Pathol 2010;34:1147–54.

80. Mazal PR, Stichenwirth M, Koller A, et al. Expression of aquaporins and PAX-2 compared to CD10 and cytokeratin 7 in renal neoplasms: a tissue microarray study. Mod Pathol 2005;18: 535–40.

81. Ozcan A, Shen SS, Hamilton C, et al. PAX 8 expression in non-neoplastic tissues, primary tumors, and metastatic tumors: a comprehensive immunohistochemical study. Mod Pathol 2011; 24:751–64.

82. Avery AK, Beckstead J, Renshaw AA, et al. Use of antibodies to RCC and CD10 in the differential diagnosis of renal neoplasms. Am J Surg Pathol 2000;24:203–10.

83. McGregor DK, Khurana KK, Cao C, et al. Diagnosing primary and metastatic renal cell carcinoma: the use of the monoclonal antibody 'Renal Cell Carcinoma Marker'. Am J Surg Pathol 2001; 25:1485–92.

84. Liu Z, Ma W, Li H, et al. Clinicopathological and prognostic features of primary clear cell carcinoma of the liver. Hepatol Res 2008;38: 291–9.

85. Jakate S, Yabes A, Giusto D, et al. Diffuse cirrhosis-like hepatocellular carcinoma: a clinically and radiographically undetected variant mimicking cirrhosis. Am J Surg Pathol 2010;34:935–41.

86. Salomao M, Yu WM, Brown RS Jr, et al. Steatohepatitic hepatocellular carcinoma (SH-HCC): a distinctive histological variant of HCC in hepatitis C virus-related cirrhosis with associated NAFLD/NASH. Am J Surg Pathol 2010;34:1630–6.

87. Jain D, Nayak NC, Saigal S. Hepatocellular carcinoma in nonalcoholic fatty liver cirrhosis and

alcoholic cirrhosis: risk factor analysis in liver transplant recipients. Eur J Gastroenterol Hepatol 2012; 24:840–8.

88. Salomao M, Remotti H, Vaughan R, et al. The steatohepatitic variant of hepatocellular carcinoma and its association with underlying steatohepatitis. Hum Pathol 2012;43:737–46.

89. Prokurat A, Kluge P, Kosciesza A, et al. Transitional liver cell tumors (TLCT) in older children and adolescents: a novel group of aggressive hepatic tumors expressing beta-catenin. Med Pediatr Oncol 2002;39:510–8.

90. Wood L, Heaphy C, Daniel H, et al. CAP carcinoma: a distinct subtype of hepatocellular carcinoma with unique morphologic and molecular features. Abstract at the United States and Canadian Academy of Pathology Annual Meeting. Vancouver, 2012:March 17–23.

Index

Note: Page numbers of article titles are in **boldface** type.

Surgical Pathology 6 (2013) 385–389
http://dx.doi.org/10.1016/S1875-9181(13)00044-5
1875-9181/13/$ – see front matter © 2013 Elsevier Inc. All rights reserved.

Moving?

Make sure your subscription moves with you!

To notify us of your new address, find your **Clinics Account Number** (located on your mailing label above your name), and contact customer service at:

Email: journalscustomerservice-usa@elsevier.com

800-654-2452 (subscribers in the U.S. & Canada)
314-447-8871 (subscribers outside of the U.S. & Canada)

Fax number: 314-447-8029

Elsevier Health Sciences Division
Subscription Customer Service
3251 Riverport Lane
Maryland Heights, MO 63043

*To ensure uninterrupted delivery of your subscription, please notify us at least 4 weeks in advance of move.

Printed and bound by CPI Group (UK) Ltd, Croydon, CR0 4YY

03/10/2024

01040347-0017